My Aspartame Experiment
Report from a Private Citizen

Victoria Inness-Brown, M.A.
aspartameexperiment.com

Writers Without Borders
DBA Writing by Design
Jamul CA 91935

Black & White Edition Version 1.0

Library of Congress Cataloging-in-Publication Data
Victoria Inness-Brown, M.A.
My Aspartame Experiment: Report from a Private Citizen

ISBN-1-4392-1046-2

1. Food. 2. Diet. 3. Nutrition. 4. Food additives. 5. Health. 6. Disease.
7. Pharmaceuticals. 8. Medical studies. 9. Politics.

April 2010

Cover and book design, photos by Victoria Inness-Brown, M.A.
Edited by Sally Altman, Damien Andrews, Gini Energy, Cher Gilmore, and Lalchumi Ralte

Printed in the United States of America
For additional copies, go to aspartameexperiment.com.

Contents

Notes

Dedication

Many have claimed to have suffered extreme ill effects from ingesting aspartame, only to have family and friends disbelieve that aspartame was the cause. Many have devoted their lives to removing aspartame from the market, often at great personal cost. I dedicate this report to you.

And I dedicate this report to my great-aunt Julia, whose life served as an inspiration to us all; to my father Hugh, whose love taught me that we can heal almost anything; to my mother Muriel, who taught me to think for myself; to my family and friends, whose support and love have so greatly enriched my life; to my friend Dr. Norm Sakow, without whose inspiration this project would never have taken place; and finally to Richard, who opened my eyes as he gave his life in service to his country.

—Victoria Inness-Brown, M.A.

Notes

"I was talking to my neighbor last evening.... He is a thirty something man that consumes a relatively good diet, but also consumes large quantities of a popular drink sweetened with aspartame.... He is having some serious health problems; serious digestion problems. (He's) on morphine for pain, he has passed out before. He has been under the care of several doctors, but he keeps getting worse ... could it be that aspartame is causing his problems?"[1]

—*Name withheld*

"Aspartame, because it is a poison that affects protein synthesis, because it affects how the synapse operates in the brain, and because it affects DNA, can affect numerous organs, so you can get a lot of different symptoms that seem unconnected."

"Again, it's this variability in your sensitivity to toxins. Some people may notice very little if anything. A majority of people will have one of a number of symptoms, because we know that the aspartame, because it is a poison that affects protein synthesis, because it affects how the synapse operates in the brain, and because it affects DNA, can affect numerous organs, so you can get a lot of different symptoms that seem unconnected."[2]

—*Dr. Russell Blaylock*

This report documents an experiment I did as a private citizen, where I administered the artificial sweetener aspartame (in the form of NutraSweet mixed with water) to 60 rats (30 male, 30 female) between May 2002 and November 2004. Another 48 rats (24 male, 24 female) were used as controls.

> **Note: In November 2009, aspartame was rebranded AminoSweet by leading manufacturer, Ajinomoto. According to the company, "The name AminoSweet is appealing and memorable. It reflects that Amino-Sweet comes from the same amino acids that are abundant in the food we eat every day."[3] The safety of consuming high concentrations of aspartame's isolated amino acids aspartic acid and phenylalanine is discussed in this report. Please see the index for listings.**

Family members were heavy diet soda drinkers

Aspartame has been the subject of hundreds of experiments. So why did I undertake another one? Several years ago I became concerned about the health of family members who were drinking large amounts of diet soda containing aspartame. I was worried that they were consuming a chemical that could one day lead to their painful and early deaths—or worse, a walking death due to Alzheimer's, Parkinson's, or some other debilitating long-term illness brought on by aspartame.

Though this report does not focus on those neurological illnesses, neurosurgeon Russell Blaylock, MD, studied the causes of those diseases for over 20 years after his father passed on from Parkinson's. Blaylock's theories about neurotoxins such as aspartame and monosodium glutamate (MSG) are eloquently described and beautifully illustrated by Blaylock in his book, *Excitotoxins, the Taste that Kills.*[4]

Convinced by the Bressler report

While researching problems associated with aspartame, I came across *The Bressler Report,*[5] which was written by an auditor working for the U.S. Food and Drug Administration (FDA). The report describes the extensive analysis performed by Jerome Bressler, MD, on an aspartame-related study undertaken by G.D. Searle & Company, a pharmaceutical corporation founded in 1888 in Skokie, Illinois. Searle is the company that first marketed aspartame, and conducted the study using diketopiperazine (DKP), the most prevalent breakdown component of aspartame.

In his report, Dr. Bressler mentions numerous instances where Searle lacked forthrightness in reporting negative results to the FDA. For example, it states that tumors were removed and rats returned to the study without the tumors or surgery being reported to the FDA. One rat was even documented as dead, and then alive, and then dead again. Because most data related to Searle's aspartame studies was under FDA seal at Searle during the time of the Bressler audit,[6] the fact that such incriminating information remained made me believe that Searle's real test results were far worse than the negative findings identified within *The Bressler Report*. While writing this report, I discovered that my belief appeared to be substantiated. According to the website, www.dorway.com:

"(Dr. Bressler) admitted the studies on aspartame were so bad that when his report was retyped, the FDA removed the worst 20 percent. So, as bad as this report is, it was originally worse."

"In a conversation with Dr. Betty Martini, Dr. H. J. Roberts and Dr. Russell Blaylock, (Dr. Bressler) admitted the studies on aspartame were so bad that when his report was retyped, the FDA removed the worst 20 percent. So, as bad as this report is, it was originally worse. Dr. Roberts wrote his congressman demanding the FDA release the other 20 percent, but they refused saying it was confidential."[7]

I was struck by the number and size of the unreported growths identified in *The Bressler Report*, and became convinced that *I* might see tumors and possibly other adverse effects if I proceeded with my own aspartame experiment. After all, a 2-in. x 1.75 in. x 1 in. (5.0 cm x 4.5 cm x 2.5 cm) tumor would be hard to miss.

I wanted visual proof of aspartame's adverse effects

If I could provide visual proof of the adverse effects of aspartame, I thought it might convince my family and friends to avoid the chemical. As a technical writer, I find that visuals add power to the written word that can otherwise be easily manipulated with statistics, fabrications or high-tech mumbo-jumbo. I also felt that showing photos of adverse effects of aspartame might add credibility to the work of the undervalued individuals independently researching the adverse effects of aspartame, and add a new tool for those who have been fighting to get aspartame off the market.

1 My Aspartame Experiment

"Dr. Ralph Walton compiled a list of all controlled human and animal studies looking for the effects of aspartame. Out of 90 independently-funded studies, 83 of them found one or more problems caused by aspartame. But out of the 74 studies funded by the aspartame industry (e.g., Monsanto, G.D. Searle, etc.), every single one claimed that no problems were found. Note that some of those 'independently-funded' studies that found no effects were funded by organizations that have been shown to have been ... run by persons with close ties to the aspartame industry."[1]

—Mark Gold, health researcher

The Bressler Report motivated me to do my own rat study on the artificial sweetener aspartame from the end of May 27, 2002 through November 2004.

The Bressler Report[2] motivated me to do my own rat study on the artificial sweetener aspartame, now rebranded as AminoSweet,[3] from May 27, 2002 through November 2004. The report is FDA auditor Dr. Jerome Bressler's extensive analysis of an aspartame-related study done by G.D. Searle & Company, the original manufacturer of aspartame. For a detailed description of the chemical, see "What is Aspartame?" on page 67.

My experimental setup is shown in Figure 1-1. Not shown are the clay saucers and upside-down clay pots that served as the rats' houses.

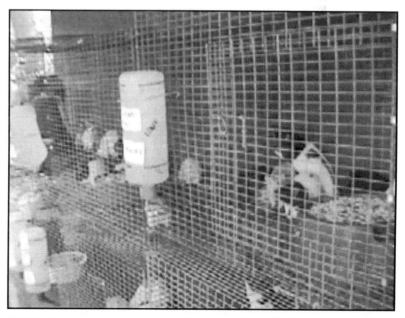

FIGURE 1-1: Experimental setup of my aspartame (AminoSweet) study

My intent was to take video of any adverse effects, and to extract photos from the video.

My intent for the experiment was to take video of any adverse effects, and to extract photos from the video. The resulting photos appear throughout this report.

I attempted to purchase pure aspartame over the Internet, but the only website I found that sold it said that it was only available to food and beverage manufacturers. Since I was prevented from purchasing pure aspartame, I mixed packets of NutraSweet (Figure 1-2) in the water I gave the rats of my experimental group.

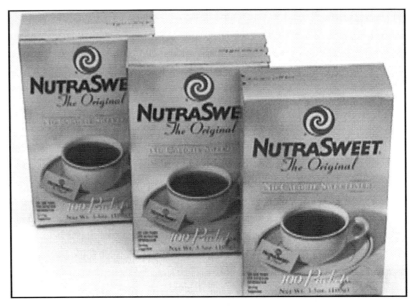

FIGURE 1-2: I mixed two packets of NutraSweet per each eight ounces of water I gave to the rats in my experimental group.

NutraSweet was the first sugarless tabletop sweetener containing aspartame that was marketed by G. D. Searle, a pharmaceutical corporation founded in 1888, originally located in Skokie, Illinois.

As my study progressed, I was amazed by the results. They contradict the studies done by the aspartame industry that consistently assure us of the safety of the additive,[4] and instead confirm the results of independent investigators that consistently show the chemical to be hazardous.[5]

To read about my experimental protocol, see Chapter 2. The results of my study are shown in Chapters 3 and 4, and my conclusion is presented in Chapter 5.

For a shocking analysis of our food, water, and air that was instigated by criticism of my experiment, see "Did I Fake My Data?" on page 91.

2

My Experimental Protocol

It is an understatement to say that as a private citizen with a minimal research budget, my protocol was unlike that of any other study I have researched.

"The FDA, which regulates both prescription and over-the-counter drugs in the United States, does not have its own facilities and funding for drug testing; rather, it issues guidelines and examines the data produced by the companies that make the medicines.... Each drug is tested under controlled conditions that don't necessarily reflect the real world."[1]

—Joe and Teresa Graedon, PhD

"Epidemiologic and experimental studies are fundamental in the identification and quantification of diffused carcinogenic risks, but they must be designed and conducted to be as powerful as possible with adequate methodology. In the case of experimental studies, it is not sufficient to follow the standard protocol used in ordinary experiments. Instead, it is necessary to conduct studies that may be defined as 'mega-experiments,' using a vast number of animals (at least 200 – 1,000 per experimental group) to express a marked difference in the variation of effects, and exposing the animals in all phases of development to allow the agent to express its full carcinogenic potential."[2]

—Dr. Morando Soffritti

This chapter provides details about my experimental protocol and compares aspects of it to similar aspects of other aspartame experiments.

Protocol summary

Table 2-1 provides a summary of my experimental protocol.

TABLE 2-1: Protocol summary for aspartame rat study

Protocol parameter	Description
Source of aspartame	NutraSweet packets (see "Diet Pepsi, aspartame or NutraSweet?" on page 5).
Form of aspartame	NutraSweet dissolved in drinking water, available 24 hours per day (see "Liquid or solid?" on page 6).
Dosage	Two packets of NutraSweet per each 8 oz. of drinking water (80 mg of aspartame per each 8 oz. of water). My males received about 34 mg/kg of aspartame per day. A 150 lb. human male ingesting 34 mg/kg of aspartame would drink about 13 12-oz. cans or 2.25 two-liter bottles of diet soda per day (see "Dosage" on page 10).

TABLE 2-1: Protocol summary for aspartame rat study

Dosage (cont.)	My females received about 45 mg/kg of aspartame per day. A 120-lb. human female ingesting 45 mg / kg of aspartame would drink about 14 12 oz. cans or 2.4 two liter bottles of diet soda per day (see "Dosage" on page 10).
Duration	Two years, five months (about 125 weeks, calculated using one month = 4.3 weeks); until the spontaneous death of the animals (see "Duration" on page 13).
Rat strain	Bred from two males, two females, each from different varieties of rats from a pet store, including one of the Sprague Dawley strain. Maintained a genetic mix throughout the breeding, avoided mating brothers and sisters, mothers and sons, fathers and daughters (see "Rat strain" on page 16).
Number of rats in study	Experimental group of 30 males, 30 females. Control group of 24 males, 24 females; for a total of 108 rats (see "Quantity of rats" on page 17).
Type of feed	Kaytee's Supreme Fortified Daily Blend for Rat & Mouse and Kaytee's Supreme Fortified Daily Blend for Hamster & Gerbil (see "Feed administered" on page 18).

Comparison studies

The studies were considered "pivotal" in the approval of aspartame by the FDA in 1981. They were done on five types of animals: mouse, rat, hamster, dog and monkey.

Table 2-2 describes five groups of long-term studies of aspartame, most of which were submitted by Searle to the FDA as proof that aspartame is safe. They were done on five types of animals: mouse, rat, hamster, dog and monkey.[3] Note that the dates on all but the last study are 1973 and 1974.

TABLE 2-2: Chronic toxicity studies of aspartame reported in 1984

Type of study	Description
Mouse	File E-75 (1974). *SC-18862: 104-Week Toxicity Study in the Mouse*, PT 984H73[4]
Rat	File E-34 (1973). *SC-18862: Two Year Toxicity Study in the Rat*, PT 838H71[5]
Hamster	File E-27 (1973). *SC-18862: 46-Week Oral Toxicity—Hamster*, PT 852S72[6]
Dog	File E-28 (1973). *SC-18862: 106-Week Oral Toxicity Study in the Dog*[7]
Monkey	"Developmental Assessment of Infant Macaques Receiving Dietary Aspartame or Phenylalanine." Published in *Aspartame: Physiology and Biochemistry; 1984*[8]

The mouse study mentioned in Table 2-2 was one of 12 safety studies submitted by Searle for validation to Universities Associated for Research and Education in Pathology (UAREP), Inc.

Note: According to the 1987 U.S. Senate Congressional Record, on August 4, 1976, G.D. Searle and FDA representatives met and resolved to allow Searle to pay the private agency UAREP $500,000 to "validate" the 12 studies.[9]

I compare aspects of the studies listed in Table 2-2 to facets of the protocol used in my study in these sections:

- "Liquid or solid?" on page 6

- "Dosage" on page 10

- "Duration" on page 13

- "Quantity of rats" on page 17

Diet Pepsi, aspartame or NutraSweet?

Because family members were addicted to diet soda, at first I wanted to put Diet Pepsi in my rats' water bottles. That idea was short lived, however. After turning a soda-filled bottle upside down and attaching it to a cage, the liquid immediately started flowing out—carbonation had pressurized the bottle—so I figured Diet Pepsi wouldn't work. It was just as well, however, because the cost of the soda would have been prohibitive over the course of the experiment.

> *Note: A 2006 Soffritti study substituted the drinking water of rats with decarbonated Coca-Cola and found it to be carcinogenic.*[10]

An Internet search revealed an aspartame supplier, but as I attempted to place the order, a message stated that only food and beverage manufacturers were permitted to purchase the chemical.

Next I decided to mix pure aspartame in their water. That approach was also short lived, however. An Internet search revealed an aspartame supplier, but as I attempted to place the order, a message stated that only food and beverage manufacturers were permitted to purchase the chemical. That practice is amazing to me, and highly questionable. Why would the company restrict its sales and thereby its profits, unless it's afraid of independent investigations into the safety of aspartame? I found those thoughts to have teeth after watching the aspartame documentary *Sweet Misery*.[11] In the film, psychiatrist Ralph G. Walton, MD, recounts his difficulty in obtaining pure aspartame for his study in the mid 1990's:

"They made the claim years ago, that they would help and support any legitimate researcher, that they would supply aspartame and be helpful in any research. I had published my anecdotal studies, and I'd written a chapter in Dr. Richard Wurtman's book, so I think the industry knew of my stands already.

> *Note: Dr. Walton wrote Chapter 18, "The Possible Role of Aspartame in Seizure Induction" in Wurtman's book.*[12]

Walton continues: *"In the mid-nineties, I wrote to the company [NutraSweet], stating that we wanted to do a double-blind study because my earlier work had indeed been anecdotal. And I pointed out that they had made the claim that they would supply the aspartame to any legitimate researcher. At that point, I was a professor at Neoucom, Northeastern Ohio Universities College of Medicine, and I think I would qualify as a legitimate researcher.*

I sent the protocol for the study to the company, and they responded that this was unnecessary research, and would not supply us with aspartame. I offered to buy the aspartame. They refused. They put up roadblocks. They made it very difficult for us to purchase aspartame. We had to go around them. We finally did get U.S. B Grade aspartame from Schweitzel, a private firm, but the point is that The NutraSweet Company made it very difficult— didn't follow through on their promise—to supply aspartame to any legitimate researcher. [They] said 'This was unnecessary, shouldn't be done, needn't be done.' They tried to block it."

Because of the difficulty *I* had purchasing pure aspartame, I decided to dissolve readily-available NutraSweet packets in water, thinking that would be more or less equivalent to administering pure aspartame. As mentioned earlier, NutraSweet was the original aspartame-based sweetener marketed by Searle.

I have since learned that other ingredients in NutraSweet may have affected the results of my study. For a discussion of what I found, see "Possible non-inert components of NutraSweet" on page 95.

Liquid or solid?

According to health researcher and writer Mark Gold, *"As soon as aspartame is dissolved in liquid it becomes unstable and begins to break down into its individual components as opposed to keeping a single stable chemical structure.... The rate of breakdown is dependent upon several factors, mainly temperature and pH."*[13]

Table 2-3 lists the forms of aspartame, either liquid or solid, used in the chronic toxicity studies reported in 1984.[14]

TABLE 2-3: Form of aspartame used in chronic toxicity studies reported in 1984

Type of study	Form of aspartame ingested
Mouse	Solid, as a "diet admix"
Rat	Solid, as a "diet admix"
Hamster	Solid "aspartame in the diet"
Dog	Solid "aspartame in the diet"
Monkey	Liquid, in formula *Similac with Iron* made by Ross Laboratories of Columbus OH; also had water available 24 hours

According to Merriam-Webster Online, *admix* is a shortened form of the word admixture, *"an element or substance added by mixing."* For example, *The Bressler Report* describes how DKP was provided as an *admixture* of rat food.

I believe I now understand why most studies were done using solid rather than liquefied aspartame. According to the authors of *Aspartame, Physiology and Biochemistry:*[15]

"Aspartame ... [is] not readily soluble in milk or water; thus it was technically difficult to achieve solution of the 3 g/kg dose of aspartame.... Every attempt was made to keep the aspartame ... in solution or in slurry form such as by hand shaking the bottles at intervals and using mechanical shaking devices on suspended bottles. Nipple holes [in the bottles] were enlarged so that the slurry of aspartame plus formula could pass through."

The difficulty of maintaining aspartame in solution is only one reason for avoiding the experimental use of liquefied aspartame. In double-blind

> *"Aspartame ... [is] not readily soluble in milk or water; thus it was technically difficult to achieve solution of the 3 g/kg dose of aspartame."*

human studies, aspartame is administered in capsules. According to Christian Tschanz, MD:[16]

"*This* [human study] *design usually requires that aspartame and placebo be administered in capsule form because aspartame's sweetness may be difficult to mask when administered in solution.*"

I had decided *not* to mix dry NutraSweet with rat food for several reasons. First, I wanted to simulate the effects of diet soda—*a liquid*. Next, NutraSweet is sold as powdered crystals that are tiny compared to the grains and alfalfa pellets comprising the food I fed my rats (see "Rat strain" on page 16). I thought that the powder would fall to the bottom of the food bowls, allowing the rats to avoid it. I knew from raising the rats that it would be tedious and difficult to calculate the dosage, because so much food ends up in the trays under their cages, mixed in with their droppings. Finally, if aspartame crystals are not completely homogenized into dry feed, they may clump, allowing rats to avoid them. Most of these factors were mentioned in *The Bressler Report,* where it described how Searle mixed dry DKP crystals in the rat food of the study audited in 1977.

> *Note: Aspartame immediately breaks down in the intestines into approximately 50% phenylalanine, 40% aspartic acid, and 10% methanol, which further breaks down into formaldehyde and formic acid.*
>
> *DKP is a breakdown component of phenylalanine, which has been studied extensively and was the subject of The Bressler Report.*

"*Liquid forms of excitotoxins, as occur in soups, gravies and diet soft drinks are more toxic than those added to solid foods ... because they are more rapidly absorbed and reach higher blood levels.*"

Aspartame is *far more potent in liquid than in solid form.* According to neuroscientist Russell L. Blaylock, MD, "*Liquid forms of excitotoxins, as occur in soups, gravies and diet soft drinks are more toxic than those added to solid foods ... because they are more rapidly absorbed and reach higher blood levels.*"[17]

Because aspartame immediately breaks down in the intestine, it does not show up in the blood after ingestion. Instead, scientists look for the individual breakdown components of aspartame.

Figure 2-1 dramatically illustrates the differences in blood levels of phenylalanine—aspartame's majority breakdown component—resulting from giving humans aspartame in solution versus capsule form. The graphs[18] in Figure 2-1 show why giving aspartame to humans in solution is much more potent than providing the chemical in capsules. The figure shows phenylalanine levels in the blood after adults have been given a single dose of aspartame in solution versus capsule form in the amount of 47 mg/kg of body weight. That amount is roughly equivalent to the aspartame received per day by the females in my study.

According to the authors of *The Clinical Evaluation of a Food Additive: Assessment of Aspartame*, capsules are usually used in human studies, because: "*aspartame's sweetness may be difficult to mask when administered in solution.*"[19] Concerns have arisen about this practice though, as voiced by the authors: "*This, however, raises additional questions because test compounds administered in capsules can produce a different pharmacokinetic profile upon absorption when compared to test compounds administered in solution. To determine the extent of this effect, we measured plasma phenylalanine concentrations in ten normal subjects given 3000 mg of aspartame in solution on one occasion and the same amount of aspartame given in capsules on another occasion. The high mean plasma phenylalanine concentrations were higher and occurred earlier when aspartame was given in solution.*"[20]

The peak average phenylalanine level from aspartame in solution increased more than 100 μM over the peak level resulting from aspartame in capsules.

Note in Figure 2-1 that the peak average phenylalanine level from aspartame in solution increased more than 100 μM over the peak level resulting from aspartame in capsules, where the peaks appear within an hour after consumption. Capsules take time to dissolve, thereby slowing the rise of phenylalanine levels.

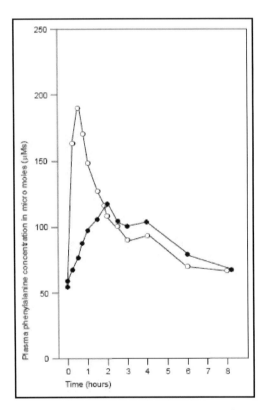

FIGURE 2-1: The vertical axis represents the mean values in micro moles (μM) of phenylalanine concentrations in the blood of normal adults administered aspartame in solution (o) versus capsules (●), at a dose of 47 mg/kg of body weight over an eight hour period.

The rapid absorption of liquid versus solid is explained by health researcher and practitioner Dr. Norm Sakow,[21] who said: "*The absorption of nutrients and chemicals into the blood stream requires that they be in liquid form. Absorption takes place through the millions of tiny villi inside the small intestine, and the villi cannot absorb anything but liquids. The ratio is about three to one—three times the nutrients are absorbed when consuming liquids compared to solids.*"

From MedTerms online medical dictionary, villi are the plural of villus, *"a tiny finger-like or hair-like projection or small vascular protrusion."* Substances absorbed by each villus pass into a capillary network that carries the substances into the blood stream.

In 1983, twice former U.S. Secretary of Defense Donald Rumsfeld, then CEO of G.D. Searle, convinced the Coca-Cola Company to switch from saccharin to NutraSweet. PepsiCo Inc. and other soft drink companies soon followed.[22] Before that, however, the National Soft Drink Association was adamantly opposed to the use of aspartame in liquids, stating that *"Aspartame is inherently, markedly, and uniquely unstable in aqueous media."* (The National Soft Drink Association has since changed its name to the American Beverage Association.[23])

> The National Soft Drink Association was adamantly opposed to the use of aspartame in liquids, stating that *"Aspartame is inherently, markedly, and uniquely unstable in aqueous media."*

Gold further states that: *"G.D. Searle, the company that originated aspartame, conducted their own stability research and forwarded their results to the FDA as part of the effort to get aspartame approved in carbonated beverages.[24] According to the information provided by G.D. Searle, when carbonated beverages are stored for eight weeks at 68°F (20°C), 11-16% of the aspartame will break down into various chemicals such as aspartic acid, phenylalanine, and significant amounts of DKP. (The breakdown into free methanol—wood alcohol—occurs at higher temperatures, and otherwise, always occurs in the small intestine after ingestion.) At 86°F (30°C) after eight weeks of storage, 38% of the aspartame will break down into its components. At 104°F (40°C), over 50% of the aspartame stored for nine weeks will break down, forming large amounts of DKP, methanol and free amino acids."*

It is important to study worst case scenarios. There is no way of knowing how aspartame-laced foods, beverages and pharmaceuticals are stored once they are packaged. We know that aspartame quickly breaks down as temperatures rise. Doesn't it make sense to study the effects of aspartame consumption where the chemical has been exposed to high temperatures? For example I've read that during Desert Storm, cases of diet soda were left out in the 125°F (52°C) Saudi Arabian sun for long periods of time. Some believe that the sodas contributed to the mysterious "Gulf War Syndrome" experienced by many veterans of that war.

From militaryspot.com: *"Gulf War Syndrome is the name given to a variety of psychological and physical symptoms suffered by veterans of the Gulf War. The symptoms have been remarkably wide-ranging, sometimes somewhat ill-defined, and distinguished by the number of theories advanced as to their origin."*

Listed as a cause of Gulf War syndrome, we find: *"Aspartame poisoning. Large quantities of aspartame sweetened diet soft drinks were provided to Gulf War troops, often times sitting in high temperature conditions. This artificial sweetener breaks down at roughly 85°F (29.5°C) into, among other things, methanol, formaldehyde, diketopiperazine and formic acid."*[25]

The aspartame in my experiment *was* exposed to a wide range of temperatures. I kept my rats outside where the average minimum and maximum temperatures range from about 42°F (6°C) to about 88°F (31°C).

Dosage

In Dr. Soffritti's mega study reported in 2005, rats were given dry aspartame mixed with dry food in concentrations of 100,000; 50,000; 10,000; 2,000; 400; 80 and 0 ppm—selected to simulate a daily intake by humans of 5,000; 2,500; 500; 100; 20; 4; or 0 mg/kg of body weight.[26]

Table 2-4 describes the dosages administered to the groups of test animals of the chronic toxicity studies introduced in Table 2-2.

TABLE 2-4: Dosages of chronic toxicity studies of aspartame reported in 1984

Type of study	Dosage
Mouse	Four groups received 0, 1000, 2000, or 4000 mg/kg of aspartame per body weight per day.
Rat	Five groups received 0, 1000, 2000, 4000, or 8000 mg/kg.
Hamster	Five groups received 0, 1000, 2000, 4000, or 12000 mg/kg.
Dog	Four groups received 0, 1000, 2000, or 4000 mg/kg.
Monkey[27]	Four groups received 0, 1000, 2000 or 3000 mg/kg.

I started by mixing a packet of NutraSweet in each eight ounces of their water.

For my experiment, I wanted to observe what would happen to rats receiving a relatively small amount of the chemical. I started by mixing a packet of NutraSweet in each eight ounces of their drinking water. After two weeks, however, I tasted the mixture, and it wasn't sweet, so I added another packet per eight ounces of water, and continued giving them two packets per eight ounces of water throughout the rest of the study. See Figure 2-2.

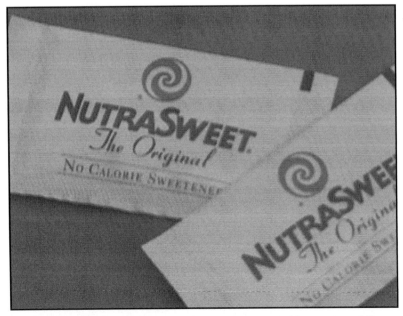

FIGURE 2-2: My rats received NutraSweet in their drinking water, at the rate of two packets per each 8 oz. of water.

According to a report on the website of the National Institutes of Health, a packet of aspartame-based sweetener such as NutraSweet contains 40 mg of aspartame,[28] and therefore two packets contain 80 mg. The aspartame administered to my rats was therefore equivalent to (80 mg/oz.) / (8 oz. water) = 10 mg/oz.

A 12-oz. diet soda has about 180 mg of aspartame, equivalent to about 4.5 packets of NutraSweet.

To put these numbers into perspective, the National Cancer Institute website states that a 12-oz. diet soda contains about 180 mg of aspartame,[29] or about (180 mg) / (40 mg / pack of NutraSweet) = 4.5 packs of NutraSweet. Diet soda therefore has approximately (180 mg) / (12 oz.) = 15 mg/oz. of aspartame. Therefore 8 oz. of diet soda has about 8 x 15 mg = 120 mg of aspartame. Since each 8 oz. of drinking water in my experiment contained about 80 mg of aspartame, the aspartame was equivalent to about 80 mg / 120 mg = 0.67 = 67%—or two-thirds the aspartame contained in 8 oz. of diet soda. The aspartame received by my rats was therefore equivalent to receiving about two-thirds of their daily fluid as diet soda and the remainder as water.

> *Note: Since I started this experiment, new kinds of diet soda have been concocted without aspartame, such as those containing Splenda. All reference to diet soda in this discussion, however, assumes that it contains aspartame unless otherwise stated.*

I have read testimonials from people who drank only liquids containing aspartame and ate multiple foods containing aspartame, so I believe that my approach was reasonable.

I neither weighed my rats nor measured their water intake on a regular basis. That was one of my failings in not having enough time or money for that level of research. I therefore substituted data for those measurements from the 2005 Soffritti study[30] in my calculation of the mg/kg of aspartame received by my rats as summarized in Table 2-5.

TABLE 2-5: Calculating the average daily intake of aspartame

Parameter	Male	Female
Average weight of rats[a]	500 g (0.5 kg; 1.1 lb.)	300 g (0.3 kg; 0.66 lb.)
Average daily H_2O intake in oz.[b]	50 ml (1.69 oz.)	40 ml (1.35 oz.)
Aspartame per oz. of H_2O intake	80 mg asp / 8 oz. H_2O = 10 mg / oz.	80 mg asp / 8 oz. H_2O = 10 mg / oz.
Average daily aspartame intake in mg.	(10 mg / oz. H_2O) x (1.69 oz.) = 16.9 mg	(10 mg / oz. H_2O) x (1.35 oz.) = 13.5 mg
Average daily aspartame intake in mg / kg	16.9 mg / 0.5 kg = 33.8 mg / kg	13.5 mg / 0.3 kg = 45 mg / kg

a. From 2005 Soffritti study
b. From 2005 Soffritti study

Of course, it would have been more exact and possibly revealing if I had regularly weighed the rats and measured their water intake. However, scientifically speaking, I feel it is reasonable to use those measurements from another study.

Each day my male rats ingested about 34 mg of aspartame per kg of body weight in their drinking water—their sole source of liquids. The females ingested about 45 mg/kg.

From the bottom row of Table 2-5, we see that my males received about 33.8 or 34 mg/kg/day of aspartame, while my females received about 45 mg/kg/day. Obviously the females, though smaller, drank more of the mixture per body weight than the males. That may partially explain why they developed more problems than the males, as shown in Chapters 3 and 4. See the discussion of this issue in "Why so many tumors in my females on aspartame" on page 93.

How many cans and two-liter bottles of diet soda would a human male or female need to ingest to receive an equivalent amount of aspartame as that ingested by my male and female rats?

If a 150 lb. (68 kg) human male ingests 34 mg/kg of aspartame per day, then the amount of aspartame he gets = (34 mg / kg / day) x (68 kg) = 2312 mg / day. A 12 oz. can of diet soda contains about 180 mg of aspartame. The equivalent amount of diet soda ingested by our male is therefore about (2312 mg) / (180 mg / 12 oz.) = 154.13 oz. per day. This is equivalent to about (154.13 oz.) / 12 oz. / can = 12.84 rounded to 13 cans, or about (154.13 oz.) / (68.48 oz. / two liter bottle) = 2.25 two-liter bottles of diet soda per day.

If a 120 lb. (54.5 kg) human female ingests 45 mg/kg of aspartame per day, then the total amount she ingests is (45 mg/kg) x (54.5 kg) = 2452.5 mg / day. The amount of diet soda required to reach this level of aspartame consumption is about (2452.5 mg x 12 oz.) / (180 mg) = 163.5 oz. of diet soda. This is equivalent to about (163.5 oz.) / 12 oz. / can = 13.63 rounded to 14 cans, or about (163.5 oz.) / (68.48 oz. / two liter bottle) = 2.4 two-liter bottles of diet soda per day.

I have met people who consume more aspartame than this each day. One is Father Joe Carroll, President of the St. Vincent de Paul Village homeless assistance agency in San Diego. In November, 2008 Father Joe received an award at a meeting of the California Medical Board where I spoke briefly about my work. At that time, he said he drank about 20 diet sodas per day.

According to the Aspartame Information Center website, the maximum allowable dose of aspartame for humans per day, called the acceptable daily intake (ADI), as set by the FDA, is 50 mg/kg.[31] The website states that the ADI is "*a very conservative estimate of the amount of a sweetener that can safely be consumed on a daily basis over a person's lifetime.*"

Based on the ADI, Table 2-6 from that website shows the maximum allowable number of servings per day of various aspartame-containing products for adults and children.

TABLE 2-6: Maximum servings per day for adults and children

Aspartame-containing product	Approximate number of servings per day to reach the ADI	
	Adult (150 lb., 68 kg)	Child (50 lb., 23 kg)
Carbonated soft drink	20 12-oz. servings (20 cans)	6 12-oz. servings (6 cans)
Powdered soft drink	33 8-oz. servings	11 8-oz. servings

TABLE 2-6: Maximum servings per day for adults and children

Gelatin	42 4-oz. servings	14 4-oz. servings
Tabletop sweetener	97 packets	32 packets

Note in Table 2-6 that the FDA claims it is safe for a 150 lb. human adult (male or female) to drink up to of 20 12-oz. cans of diet soda per day. So the equivalent amount that a human male or female would receive during my experiment would be less than the ADI.

How much less? The equivalent a 150-lb. (68 kg) human male would receive in my experiment is 13 cans of diet soda per day, which is $13/20 = 0.65 = 65\%$ of the ADI. The equivalent a 120 lb. (54.5 kg) human female would receive in my experiment is 14 cans per day, which is $14/20 = 0.70 = 70\%$ of the ADI.

Duration

Rather than sacrificing my rats at some point in my experiment, as is done in many studies, I chose to allow my rats to live out their natural lives. After I decided to proceed with the experiment, I communicated about it through e-mail with Robert Cohen, an animal-rights activist with an educational website and e-mail list about the hazards of consuming dairy products.[32]

Robert was a close associate of now-deceased Dave Rietz, webmaster of the extensive anti-aspartame site, www.dorway.com. As an animal rights advocate, Robert sent me a heated message about doing an animal experiment. He then forwarded my message to Dave, another animal rights activist, who also let me have it in no uncertain terms about my project.

But I was determined to proceed. My love for my family and concern for others preempted my concern for the relatively few rats that would participate in my experiment, when compared to the 200,000,000 people worldwide estimated to consume the additive.[33]

We are the rats of the pharmaceutical and chemical companies that liberally spread their synthetic chemicals worldwide, with no one fully understanding the long-term adverse effects.

Through my research, I have come to the conclusion that *most*, if not *all* food additives and pharmaceuticals are not fully understood when they go to market. In my opinion, *we are the rats of the pharmaceutical and chemical companies* that liberally spread their synthetic chemicals worldwide, with no one fully understanding the long-term adverse effects—especially the complex interactions from intermixing thousands of toxic chemicals within the plant and animal kingdoms sustaining our planet.

I felt that if we could unquestionably show the damage done by aspartame, then the suffering of my rats would be outweighed by the benefits to the many that might be helped as a result.

I have always felt sorry for lab animals myself, so after I was criticized by Robert and Dave, I determined that I would *not* sacrifice my animals.

When showing photos of my study to a friend who runs a lab, she said she would have put down the animals that had become so diseased. I thought about that, but then I remembered my promise to allow them to live out their natural lives. In addition, it seemed necessary to observe how extreme their diseases would become before they died. Also, it seems to me that veterinary intervention would have affected the outcome of the experiment.

After the recent passing of my great aunt and natural father and witnessing their tremendous will to live in spite of the pain of their illnesses; and after listening to a radio show on PBS about dying and the will to live, I believe that most people, no matter how sick and physically devastated they are, have a strong will to live, often until moments before death. I'd like to think that my rats felt the same way, and I honor them for their sacrifice.

I put NutraSweet in their water starting on May 27, 2002, and the last two rats died in early November 2004. The experiment lasted a total of two years, five months.

Italian scientist Dr. Morando Soffritti calls his experiments *lifetime mega experiments*.[34] During each experiment, his team makes observations of thousands of rats until their "spontaneous deaths."

"One of the most important issues in environmental and industrial carcinogenesis is how to deal with diffused carcinogenic risks to which most of the planet's population may be exposed."

Soffritti is driven by the belief that: "*One of the most important issues in environmental and industrial carcinogenesis is how to deal with diffused carcinogenic risks* [such as those posed by aspartame], *to which most of the planet's population may be exposed. These carcinogenic risks are represented by a) agents slightly carcinogenic at any dose; b) low or extremely low doses of a carcinogenic agents of any kind; or c) mixtures of small doses of carcinogenic agents.*"[35]

Soffritti reasons that most cancer occurs in the last third of a person's lifespan, and calls it poor laboratory practice when: "*most studies sacrifice their animals at a maximum of 110 weeks* [two years, six weeks] *of age.*"

Soffritti further states that "*The Ramazzini study design closely mirrors the human condition in which persons may be exposed to agents in the industrial and general environments from embryonic life until natural death. Since 80% of cancer is diagnosed in humans over the age of 55, it is of paramount importance to observe how an agent affects laboratory animals in the last third of their lives.*"

Since 1984, the Ramazzini Foundation, in its Cancer Research Center at Bentivoglio, Italy, has completed five mega experiments under Soffritti,[36] and his results have provided the scientific basis for changes in international regulations numerous times over the past 30 years.[37] One found the fuel additive MTBE to be carcinogenic. The results were readily accepted by the scientific community and several states banned the use of the additive.[38]

In total, the Ramazzini Foundation has studied over 200 chemicals. In addition to aspartame and MTBE, it has found the following chemicals to be carcinogens: vinyl chloride, benzene, formaldehyde, gasoline and its components, and some pesticides.[39] It is interesting to note that formaldehyde is a breakdown component of aspartame, and may partly explain the tumors in my study.

Continuing our analysis of the aspartame toxicity studies listed in Table 2-2, Table 2-7 shows the duration of each type of study.

TABLE 2-7: Duration of chronic toxicity studies of aspartame reported in 1984

Type of study	Duration
Mouse	110 weeks (2 years, 6 weeks)
Rat	104 weeks (2 years)
Hamster	46 weeks
Dog	106 weeks (2 years, 2 weeks)
Monkey	9 months

I did not have the financial wherewithal or knowledge to experiment with thousands of rats. However, in my 2 year, 5 month study, I observed the final stages of life of both experimental and control rats, and found that many of my documented adverse results took place in the last third of their lives.

I have been severely criticized, even losing a friendship because of my experiment. I was told that what I did was morally and ethically wrong. The person who criticized me is so immersed in the righteousness of the pharmaceutical companies that I found myself defenseless against his angry words.

"Aspartame has been safely consumed for nearly a quarter of a century and is one of the most thoroughly studied food ingredients, with more than 200 scientific studies confirming its safety."

The aspartame industry touts that more than 200 studies have demonstrated the safety of the additive. A typical statement is: "*Aspartame has been safely consumed for nearly a quarter of a century and is one of the most thoroughly studied food ingredients, with more than 200 scientific studies confirming its safety.*"[40]

Table 2-8 shows the durations of various human studies whose descriptions were published in 1996 by then-aspartame manufacturer Monsanto. Each row of Table 2-8 represents a set of studies. The Maximum Duration column shows the duration of the longest running study within each set. Assuming that the average human lifespan is 70 years, the third column represents the percentage of a lifespan during which the tests were executed.

TABLE 2-8: Duration of human studies proving the safety of aspartame in 1996

Study	Maximum duration	Percentage of 70 year lifespan
"Metabolism and Pharmacokinetics of Radio-labeled Aspartame in Normal Subjects"[41]	7 days	(7 days) / (25550 days) = 0.03%
"Effects of Aspartame Ingestion on Plasma Aspartate, Phenylalanine, and Methanol Concentrations in Normal Adults"[42]	24 hours	(24 hrs) / (613200 hrs) = 0.004%
"Effects of Aspartame Ingestion on Plasma Aspartate, Phenylalanine, and Methanol Concentrations in Potentially Sensitive Populations"[43]	24 weeks	(24 weeks) / (3640 weeks) = 0.66%
"Safety Evaluation in Pregnancy"[44]	6 months	(6 months) / (840 months) = 0.71%
"Tolerance in Healthy Adults and Children"[45]	27 weeks	(27 weeks) / (3640 weeks) = 0.74%
"Tolerance in Individuals with Diabetes"[46]	18 weeks	(18 weeks) / (3640 weeks) = 0.49%

TABLE 2-8: Duration of human studies proving the safety of aspartame in 1996

"Tolerance in PKU Heterozygotes"[47]	21 weeks	(21 weeks) / (3640 weeks) = 0.58%
"Tolerance in Individuals with Renal (Kidney) Disease"[48]	18 weeks	(18 weeks) / (3640 weeks) = 0.49%
"Tolerance in Individuals with Liver Disease"[49]	7 days	(7 days) / (25550 days) = 0.03%

> *Note: 70 years = (70 years) x (12 months/year) = 840 months = (70 years) x (52 weeks/year) = 3640 weeks = (70 years) x (365 days/year) = 25550 days = (24 hours/day) x (25550 days) = 613200 hours.*

Column 3 shows that the durations of these studies were each an extremely small percentage of the human lifespan. In fact, *each of these human studies was administered for less than 1% of an average person's lifetime.*

To me it is unconscionable that the aspartame industry would do so many experiments of such short durations, and then claim they show the additive to be harmless.

In my opinion, there is no way that such brief studies could prove the safety of the chronic use of the chemical. I feel that the animals involved in all aspartame industry studies were sacrificed to provide false security for marketing a highly toxic chemical to the unsuspecting public.

Rat strain

Most pharmaceutical company-sponsored studies are done on rats or mice that are genetically identical. I'm not sure about the colony of Sprague-Dawley rats used in the Soffritti studies. However, according to a friend who runs a rabbit and mouse lab for a local biotech company, "*There are vendors that have specific strains of rats ... [that] are genetically identical. They've gone through 30 generations of brother and sister in-bred mating.*"

This concept seems counter-intuitive to me. How do these strains of rats represent the general population? Dr. Jay Phelan is a Harvard and Yale-educated biology professor specializing in evolutionary genetics at UCLA. According to Dr. Phelan in his remarkable book *Mean Genes,* co-written with Dr. Terry Burnhan:

"*Almost all animals avoid mating with close relatives because it makes for bad babies. From mice to monkeys, animals are reluctant to have offspring with siblings.*"[50]

I bought rats at a local pet store and bred them for my experiment. I purchased rats of different colors to get a genetic variety. I also attempted to breed rats that were not brothers and sisters, because the biology classes that I took said that in-breeding can cause genetic mutations.

Think about it. Which group more approximates the general population? How does a group of rats resulting from unnatural incestuous relationships

To me it is unconscionable that the aspartame industry would do so many experiments of such short durations, and then claim they show the additive to be harmless.

for 30 generations approximate the general human population? Humans do not generally have such relationships—especially for 30 generations. Also, if the rats in the control and study groups must be identical to have valid statistics, does that mean that all human studies, where almost no one is genetically identical to anyone else, are invalid?

When I posed these questions to author Jay Phelan after tracking him down on the Internet, he sent me the following message:

"I think that using completely inbred strains of animals for lab experimentation is definitely not the best practice. The process of inbreeding creates a lot of genetic problems for a population that can cause them not simply to be more prone to disease but to be susceptible to a variety of usually rare health problems. Moreover, different strains are susceptible to different illnesses so the research results may vary more than researchers expect dependent upon which strain(s) they have used. And, as you point out, humans are relatively outbred so it is best to choose an experimental system with a similarly heterozygous genome."[51]

"I think that using completely inbred strains of animals for lab experimentation is definitely not the best practice."

Quantity of rats

As mentioned earlier, I raised all rats for my study except for the initial four that survived out of the eight I purchased for the experiment.

Out of a total of 108 rats in my study, there were 60 in the experimental aspartame group—30 males and 30 females. There were 48 in the control group—24 males and 24 females. Because I became attached to the older rats, I placed the younger ones in the experimental group.

Continuing our running analysis of the toxicity studies of aspartame listed in Table 2-2, Table 2-9 shows the quantity of animals in each study.

TABLE 2-9: Number of animals in chronic toxicity studies of aspartame

Type of study	Quantity of animals in study
Mouse	Three groups of 36 male and 36 female (72 per dose group) = 216 experimental mice + 72 male and 72 female control mice = 360 mice
Rat	Four groups of 40 male and 40 female rats (80 per dose group) = 320 rats + 60 male and 60 female control rats = 440 rats
Hamster	Four groups of five male and five female hamsters (10 per dose group) = 40 hamsters + 10 male and 10 female control hamsters = 60 hamsters
Dog	Four groups of five male and five female (10 per dose group) = 40 dogs
Monkey	Four groups of four infant monkeys (four per dose group) = 16 monkeys + four monkeys as controls = 20 monkeys

While the mouse and rat studies contained significantly more animals than mine, the hamster, dog, and monkey studies contained significantly fewer animals.

While the mouse and rat studies contained significantly more animals than mine, the hamster, dog, and monkey studies contained significantly fewer animals. Though Morando Soffritti would probably consider that the number of rats in my study invalidate it as a "mega experiment," considering the small number of animals in numerous studies accepted by the FDA, I believe that the number of rats in my study is sufficient to support the legitimacy of the results compared to the other experiments accepted by the FDA as proof of aspartame's safety.

Feed administered

I fed my animals Kaytee's[52] Supreme Fortified Daily Blend for Rat & Mouse or Kaytee's Supreme Fortified Daily Blend for Hamster & Gerbil from a local feed store, along with occasional fruits and greens and well water to drink. Table 2-10 shows the contents of Kaytee's Rat & Mouse feed. Table 2-11 shows the contents of Kaytee's Hamster & Gerbil feed.

TABLE 2-10: Ingredients and nutritional analysis of Kaytee's Rat & Mouse feed

Ingredients	Rolled corn, rolled oat groats, rolled barley, ground corn, dehulled soybean meal, wheat middlings, ground wheat, dehydrated alfalfa meal, meat meal, sunflower seeds, peanuts, corn gluten meal, cane molasses, vegetable oil, poultry meal, fish meal, salt, beet pulp, calcium carbonate, brewers dried yeast, iron oxide, lignin sulfonate, dicalcium phosphate, DL-methionine, vitamin A supplement, choline chloride, ferrous carbonate, manganous oxide, zinc oxide, riboflavin supplement, vitamin B12, vitamin E, ethoxyquin (a preservative), copper sulfate, niacin, menadione sodium bisulfite complex (source of vitamin K), cholecalciferol (source of vitamin D3), calcium pantothenate, pyridoxine hydrochloride, thiamine mononitrate, calcium iodate, biotin, folic acid, cobalt carbonate, sodium selenite.	
Nutritional analysis	Crude protein (minimum)	15%
	Crude fat (minimum)	5.0%
	Crude fiber (maximum)	9.0%
	Moisture (maximum)	12.0%

TABLE 2-11: Ingredients and nutritional analysis of Kaytee's Hamster & Gerbil feed

Ingredients	Rolled corn, rolled oat groats, rolled barley, sunflower, soybean meal, peanuts, ground corn, ground wheat, ground oats, wheat middlings, dehydrated alfalfa meal, cane molasses, calcium carbonate, fish meal, salt, brewers dried yeast, lignin sulfonate, dicalcium phosphate, DL-methionine, iron oxide, vitamin A supplement, choline chloride, riboflavin supplement, vitamin B12 supplement, vitamin E supplement, ethoxyquin (a preservative), copper sulfate, ferrous carbonate, manganous oxide, zinc oxide, niacin, menadione sodium bisulfite complex (source of vitamin K), cholecalciferol (source of vitamin D3), calcium pantothenate, pyridoxine hydrochloride, thiamine mononitrate, calcium iodate, biotin, folic acid, cobalt carbonate, sodium selenite.	
Nutritional analysis	Crude protein (minimum)	14%
	Crude fat (minimum)	4.0%
	Crude fiber (maximum)	10.0%
	Moisture (maximum)	12.0%

3 Resulting Tumors

"It is physiologically impossible for aspartame to cause cancer.... Long-term and lifetime tests in rats and mice with extremely large amounts of aspartame showed no evidence of brain tumors or any cancer associated with aspartame."

"It is physiologicaldicly impossible for aspartame to cause cancer.... Long-term and lifetime tests in rats and mice with extremely large amounts of aspartame showed no evidence of brain tumors or any cancer associated with aspartame."[1]

—International Food Information Council (IFIC) Foundation; *"IFIC is supported primarily by the broad-based food, beverage, and agricultural industries."*[2]

"Aspartame ... was administered with feed to male and female Sprague-Dawley rats (100-150/sex/group), 8 weeks-old at the start of the experiment, at concentrations of 100,000; 50,000; 10,000; 2,000; 400; 80 and 0 ppm. Treatment lasted until spontaneous death of the animals.... The first results (show) that aspartame, in our experimental conditions, causes a statistically significant, dose-related increase in lymphomas...."[3]

—Dr. Morando Soffritti, Fiorella Belpoggi, Davide Degli Esposti, and Luca Lambertini

Of all the effects of aspartame ingestion that I observed during my experiment, I found tumors to be the most frequent, often shocking, adverse effect. The sheer size and number of tumors in the aspartame group was astounding. I feel that there may be other reasons why the tumors were so plentiful and huge. For a discussion of my findings, see "Why so many tumors in my females on aspartame?" on page 93.

In his seven-year rat study on aspartame, Dr. Morando Soffritti from Bologna, Italy found aspartame to be associated with unusually high rates of lymphomas (cancer of the lymph glands), leukemias and other cancers. The study involved 1,900 laboratory rats that received doses of aspartame that started at rates equivalent to a 150-pound person drinking four to five 20-ounce bottles of diet soda per day.

In an article from the September 2007 issue of *Environmental Health Perspectives*, Soffritti states:

"In a previous study conducted at the Cesare Maltoni Cancer Research Center of the European Ramazzini Foundation (CMCRC/ERF), we demonstrated for the first time that aspartame (APM) is a multipotent carcinogenic agent when various doses are administered with feed to Sprague-Dawley rats from 8 weeks of age throughout the life span.

"[In a subsequent mega experiment] we studied groups of 70-95 male and female Sprague-Dawley rats administered APM (2,000, 400, or 0 ppm) with feed from the 12th day of fetal life until natural death.

"Our results show:

"a) A significant dose-related increase of malignant tumor-bearing animals in males ... particularly in the group treated with 2,000 ppm APM

"b) A significant increase in incidence of lymphomas/leukemias in males treated with 2,000 ppm ... and a significant dose-related increase in incidence of lymphomas/leukemias in females ... particularly in the 2,000-ppm group.

"c) A significant dose-related increase in incidence of mammary cancer in females ... particularly in the 2,000-ppm group.

> *"The results of this carcinogenicity bioassay ... reinforce the first experimental demonstration of APM's multipotential carcinogenicity at a dose level close to the acceptable daily intake for humans."*

"Conclusions. The results of this carcinogenicity bioassay confirm and rein-force the first experimental demonstration of APM's multipotential carcino-genicity at a dose level close to the acceptable daily intake for humans. Furthermore, the study demonstrates that when life-span exposure to APM begins during fetal life, its carcinogenic effects are increased."[4]

In an apparent response to the damaging reports of the Soffritti studies pub-lished in 2005 and 2007, Ajinomoto of Japan—one of the world's largest producers of aspartame—sponsored its own safety evaluation of the artificial sweetener that has come to be known as the Magnuson 2007 review.

The conclusion of an article about the Magnuson 2007 review published in the journal *Critical Reviews in Toxicology* states that:

"Aspartame's metabolism is well understood and follows that of other com-mon foods. Aspartame consumption, even at levels much higher than that expected under typical circumstances, has virtually no impact on levels of other blood constituents such as amino acids, methanol or glucose. Aspar-tame is a well-studied sweetener whose safety is clearly documented and well established through extensive laboratory testing, animal experiments, epidemiological studies, and human clinical trials. Controlled and thorough scientific studies confirm aspartame's safety and find no credible link between consumption of aspartame at levels found in the human diet and conditions related to the nervous system and behavior, nor any other symp-tom or illness. Aspartame is well documented to be nongenotoxic [non-toxic to genes] and there is no credible evidence that aspartame is carcinogenic. Aspartame does not increase hunger in those that use it; to the contrary, studies indicate it might be an effective tool as part of an overall weight management program. Aspartame is a well-characterized, thoroughly stud-ied, high-intensity sweetener that has a long history of safe use in the food supply and can help reduce the caloric content of a wide variety of foods."[5]

Health researcher Mark Gold, however, found massive conflicts of interest in those who performed the Magnuson 2007 review. According to Gold, in a well-documented investigative report online, *"Nearly every section of the Magnuson 2007 review has research that is misrepresented and/or crucial pieces of information are left out. In addition ... readers (including medical professionals) are often not told that this review was funded by the aspar-tame manufacturer, Ajinomoto, and the reviewers had enormous conflicts of interest."*

Informa Healthcare, the parent company of the journal reporting the Magnuson 2007 study, stated in a press release that *"There were no known conflicts of interest with the sponsor* [Aji-nomoto] *or potential biases of the authors."* Yet Gold found that most of the authors had serious conflicts of interest not documented in the report.

Gold notes that Informa Healthcare, the parent company of the journal reporting the Magnuson 2007 study, stated in a press release that *"There were no known conflicts of interest with the sponsor* [Ajinomoto] *or potential biases of the authors."* Yet Gold found most authors to have serious conflicts of interest not documented in the report. For example:

- Bernadine Magnuson: the lead author of the review (for whom the study was nicknamed the "Magnuson 2007 review") was the *"Senior Scientific and Regulatory Consultant for Cantox Health Sciences International, a corporate advocacy group. Cantox (now known as Intrinsik) specializes 'in assisting clients in their efforts to develop, gain regulatory approval and market products nationally or internationally.' ... In 2002, the president of Cantox, Ian C. Munro, worked directly with NutraSweet company employees and consultants on an aspartame review where he stated: 'After 30 plus years of rigorous scientific research, it is time to put questions of aspartame safety to rest.... The continuing debate over such a non-issue only serves to divert attention and the allocation of resources from more important health issues that need to be addressed.' Bernadene Magnuson became a member of the corporate advocacy group, The Burdock Group in 2005. The Burdock Group offers its clients 'technically rigorous, comprehensive safety and regulatory management of their products.... The Burdock Group offers the highest quality consulting services for the safety and regulatory issues facing the Food and Beverage, Dietary Supplement, Cosmetics/Personal Care and Pet Food Industries. Together, we form a cohesive team that offers single-source solutions for your business's safety assessment and regulatory needs.'"*

- G. A. Burdock: is part of the Burdock Group just mentioned.

- John Doull: *"a paid consultant of Monsanto* [previous manufacturer of aspartame], *a member of the Monsanto-funded ACSH Advisory Board, and a Trustee of the Monsanto- and Ajinomoto-funded corporate research association,* [International Life Sciences Institute] *ILSI."*

- R. M. Kroes: *"joined with Ian C. Munro, the president of the Cantox Health Sciences International corporate advocacy group, to work with Monsanto to review its herbicide, glyphosate."*

- G. M. Marsh: *"had research funded by the Formaldehyde Institute, a trade association consisting of Monsanto, Dupont and other chemical companies. The Formaldehyde Institute raised money for research in an attempt to portray formaldehyde exposure in a good light. Since independent published research has shown that aspartame ingestion leads to formaldehyde accumulation in the brain, kidneys, liver and other organs and tissues, Gary Marsh's research for the Formaldehyde Institute is a serious conflict of interest."*

- Michael Pariza: *"was a scientific advisor to the industry-funded advocacy group, 'American Council on Science & Health.' According to an article in the Washington Post: 'In 1982, the American Council on Science and Health (ACSH) filed a friend-of-the-court brief in a Formaldehyde Institute lawsuit that overturned a federal ban on formaldehyde insulation.... At least a third of ACSH's funding comes from such companies as Allied Corp., Coca-Cola, the National Soft Drink Association, Colgate-Palmolive Co., Dow Chemical Canada, Dupont, Eli Lilly, Exxon, General Mills, General Foods Fund, Gulf Oil, Hershey Foods, Johnson & Johnson, Kellogg's, Monsanto Fund, Mobil Foundation, M&M/Mars, Pillsbury Foundation, Procter & Gamble, Pfizer, Shell Oil, Upjohn and Velsicol Chemical.' Michael Pariza is also a member of the Board of Trustees of the International Life Sciences Institute (ILSI), a chemical and food company research association funded by Ajinomoto, Monsanto, Coca-Cola, PepsiCo, Nestle, and many other food and chemical companies involved in the production, use and sale of aspartame.*

- Ronald Walker: *"spent seven years as the ILSI's Chairman of their Scientific Committee on Toxicology/Food Safety in Europe. As mentioned earlier, ILSI is funded by Monsanto, Ajinomoto, Coca-Cola, Pepsi Cola, etc. He was a consultant for DSM Nutritional Products, a company that sold 'Twinsweet' from Holland Sweetener Company which is a mixture of aspartame and acesulfame-k. The DSM web site contained aspartame advocacy articles written by Holland Sweetener Company. He was a consultant for Numico Beheer BV/Danone Group, a company that had a joint venture with Ajinomoto (the sponsor of this review). He is a paid consultant to the corporate public relations group, the European Food Information Council with corporate members that include Coca-Cola, PepsiCo, Dannon, Nestle, etc. Finally, he was a paid consultant for Cantox Health Sciences International. Ronald Walker wrote a glowing review of another Ajinomoto product, monosodium glutamate (MSG) for a symposium funded by an Ajinomoto managed trade group, International Glutamate Technical Committee (IGTC). He participated in another aspartame review where he claimed that aspartame was safe."*

- Gary M. Williams: *"was the Chairman of the American Health Foundation (AHF) which was funded in part by The NutraSweet Company and other companies selling aspartame-containing products. AHF Board of Directors have included representatives of PepsiCo and the National Soft Drink Association. The AHF received more than $163,000 in grants from Philip Morris.... In 1987, the AHF convened a conference,* Sweeteners: Health Effects, *where an AHF representative concluded that aspartame and other sweeteners were safe: 'It is clear from the perspective of potential cancer risk that the sweeteners described in some detail in this report are safe and wholesome, and perhaps more so, than sugar. As we noted, it is our hope that this workshop will be the basis for international recognition of this fact, so that medical research effects can be directed effectively to areas more relevant to health maintenance.' Gary Williams also joined with Ian Munro to work with Monsanto to review its herbicide, glyphosate."*[6]

Only two authors of the Magnuson 2007 review appear to be free of conflicts of interest, as Gold provided no evidence against them: P. S. Spencer from Oregon Health and Science University, Portland, Oregon, USA; and W. J. Waddell from the University of Louisville Medical School, Louisville, Kentucky, USA.

One of the studies mentioned in the Magnuson 2007 review was a massive study undertaken by the Division of Cancer Epidemiology and Genetics, Division of Cancer Control and Population Sciences, National Cancer Institute, National Institute of Health (NIH), Department of Health and Human Services (DHHS), Information Management Services, Inc., Rockville, Maryland; and the American Association of Retired Persons (AARP), Washington, District of Columbia.

According to this study:

"Background: In a few animal experiments, aspartame has been linked to hematopoietic and brain cancers. Most animal studies have found no increase in the risk of these or other cancers. Data on humans are sparse for either cancer. Concern lingers regarding this widely used artificial sweetener.

"Objective: We investigated prospectively whether aspartame consumption is associated with the risk of hematopoietic cancers or gliomas (malignant brain cancer).

"Methods: We examined 285,079 men and 188,905 women ages 50 to 71 years in the NIH-AARP Diet and Health Study cohort. Daily aspartame intake was derived from responses to a baseline self-administered food frequency questionnaire that queried consumption of four aspartame-containing beverages (soda, fruit drinks, sweetened iced tea, and aspartame added to hot coffee and tea) during the past year. Histologically confirmed incident cancers were identified from eight state cancer registries....

"Results: During over 5 years of follow-up (1995-2000), 1,888 hematopoietic cancers and 315 malignant gliomas were ascertained. Higher levels of aspartame intake were not associated with the risk of overall hematopoietic cancer (RR for 600 mg/d, 0.98; 95% CI, 0.76-1.27), glioma (RR for 400 mg/d, 0.73; 95% CI, 0.46-1.15; P for inverse linear trend = 0.05), or their subtypes in men and women.

"Conclusions: Our findings do not support the hypothesis that aspartame increases hematopoietic or brain cancer risk. (Cancer Epidemiology Biomarkers, and Prevention; 2006; 15(9); p 1654-9)"[7]

> On the surface, the AARP and NIH study mentioned in the Magnuson 2007 review looks impressive with 473,984 subjects. That is a massive number rarely seen in a single study.

On the surface, the AARP and NIH study mentioned above looks impressive with 473,984 subjects. That is a massive number rarely seen in a single study. As you investigate it, however, you'll find it has major flaws. The biggest flaw is that it was based on a food survey that was not designed to evaluate aspartame consumption.

Participants were only queried on the consumption *"of four aspartame-containing beverages (soda, fruit drinks, sweetened iced tea, and aspartame added to hot coffee and tea)."* Note that this description does not specify whether or not participants were questioned on their consumption of diet soda, diet fruit drinks, and artificially sweetened iced tea. It appears that those values were estimated. In addition, the study was highly limited regarding ingestion of aspartame, since the additive is present in over 6,000 consumables.

Regarding the validity of such a survey in general, the food frequency questionnaire itself has come into question. In another article from the same journal, Alan Kristal, Ulrike Peters, and John Potter made the statement:

"Although painful to admit, it is possible that epidemiologists have been deluded in their acceptance of food frequency questionnaires (FFQ) as the standard tool for dietary assessment in large studies of diet and cancer. The substantial limitations of FFQs have been known for some time.... However, few of us expected the astonishingly poor measurement characteristics of FFQs ... nor had we expected to learn that diet and cancer associations detected when dietary assessment is based on dietary biomarkers or food records are undetectable when based on FFQs. We are facing a crisis: hundreds of millions of dollars and many scientists' careers have been invested in studies using only FFQs to measure diet, but it is possible that these studies have not been, and will not be, able to answer many if not most questions about diet and cancer risk."[8]

> *"We are facing a crisis: hundreds of millions of dollars and many scientists' careers have been invested in studies using only FFQs to measure diet, but it is possible that these studies have not been, and will not be, able to answer many if not most questions about diet and cancer risk."*

In addition, the questionnaires of many people who may have had blood or brain cancers were thrown out of the study. From an article about the NIH-AARP Diet and Health Study we find:

"Out of 617,119 questionnaires returned, 567,169 were satisfactorily completed. We excluded ... 582 persons who had died or moved out of the study area before study entry, 52,887 persons with history of cancer ... or with only death reports of cancer."[9]

So the questionnaires of many of the people who may have had cancers due to aspartame ingestion were eliminated from the study.

Tumors in my aspartame group

My females on aspartame were hardest hit, with a phenomenal 20 out of 30 = two-thirds or 67% of them developing visible tumors as shown in the following subsection. For an in-depth analysis of possible causes, see "Why so many tumors in my females on aspartame?" on page 93. In comparison, only 7 out of 30 = 23% of my males on aspartame developed visible tumors. See "Males on aspartame with tumors" on page 34. For observations about these results, see "Females on aspartame had three times more tumors than males" on page 92.

Females in my control group also developed tumors. See "Tumors in my control group" on page 38. For a frightening analysis of possible causes, see "What may have caused my control group tumors?" on page 99.

For a complete summary of my results, see "Summary of my experimental results" on page 61.

Females on aspartame with tumors

The following subsections show various groups of females on aspartame with tumors, organized by color.

White and black females with lymph or mammary gland tumors

The females in my experiment shown in Figure 3-1 through Figure 3-3 developed apparent tumors of the lymph or mammary gland. According to a local veterinarian, when a rat develops a tumor, it is most likely malignant. According to the book, *The Rat: An Owner's Guide to a Healthy Pet*, however, "*Most growths that rats get are benign.*"[10] Since I did not have necropsies performed, we don't know which tumors were benign or malignant. However, I would not want to walk around with any of these tumors, whether benign or not.

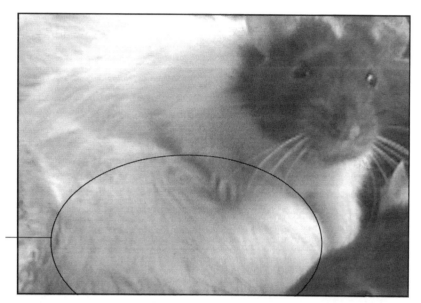

This female on aspartame often used her tumor as a pillow.

FIGURE 3-1: Female on aspartame that developed a huge tumor of the breast or lymph gland that she often used as a pillow.

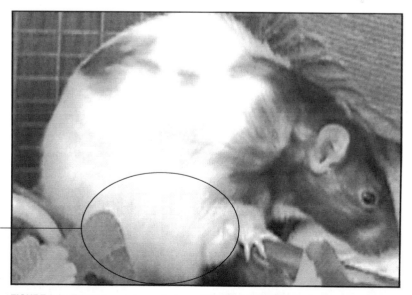

This female had an apparent lymph or mammary gland tumor on her right side.

FIGURE 3-2: Female on aspartame with an apparent lymph or mammary gland tumor.

The female in Figure 3-3 also developed an apparent lymph or mammary gland tumor. She was one of the last surviving rats of the experiment ending in November 2004.

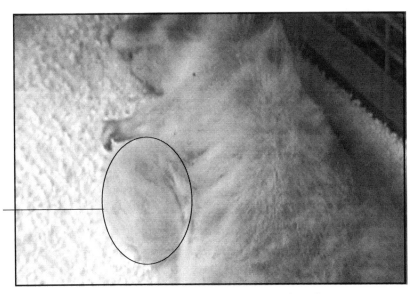

This female had an apparent lymph or mammary gland tumor near her right foreleg.

FIGURE 3-3: Female on aspartame with an apparent lymph or mammary gland tumor.

White and black females with lymph or mammary gland tumors and yellow tinged fur

In my experiment, the white and black females on aspartame shown in Figure 3-4 through Figure 3-14 had apparent lymph or mammary gland tumors. In addition, each had tinges of yellowing fur, which unfortunately is not discernible in the black-and-white version of this report. It is, however, a possible effect of aspartame. (See "Yellowing fur" on page 58.)

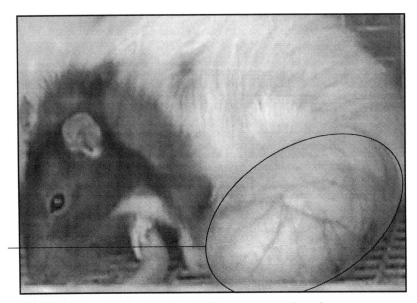

This female had an apparent lymph or mammary gland tumor near her left foreleg.

FIGURE 3-4: Female on aspartame with an apparent lymph or mammary gland tumor and yellowing fur.

The female in Figure 3-4 also had skin problems, indicated by the scabbing which is barely visible on the far-right underside of her tumor. (See "Skin disorders within my aspartame group" on page 53.) The tumor on the female in Figure 3-5 grew to gigantic proportions and appeared filled with numerous smaller tumors. Note how it almost completely surrounded her left foreleg, causing her great difficulty when walking.

The tumor on this female grew to enormous proportions and appeared filled with numerous smaller tumors.

Note how the tumor sack almost completely engulfed her left foreleg.

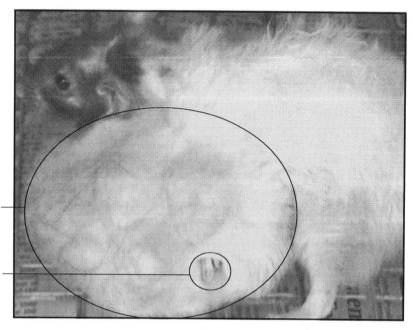

FIGURE 3-5: Female on aspartame that developed an immense lymph or mammary growth that appears subdivided into smaller tumors.

This female had an apparent lymph or mammary gland tumor near her right hind leg.

She also had a tumor on the right side of her face.

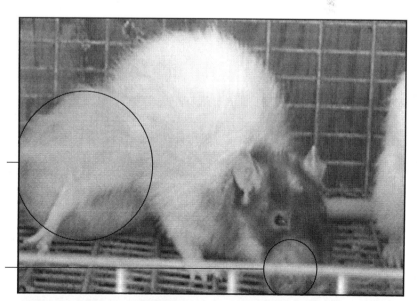

FIGURE 3-6: Female on aspartame with a tumor of the lymph or mammary gland and another on her face.

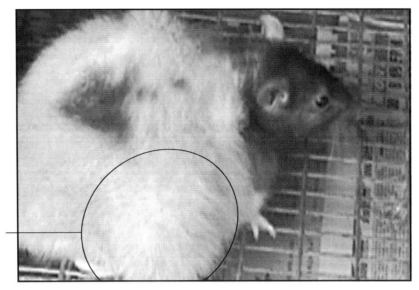

This female had an apparent lymph or mammary gland tumor near her right foreleg.

FIGURE 3-7: Aspartame female with an apparent lymph or mammary gland tumor near her right foreleg.

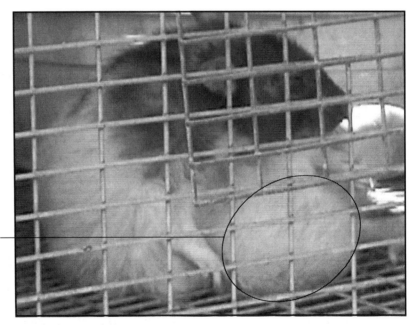

This female had an apparent tumor of the lymph or mammary gland near her right hind leg.

She also appeared to have bleeding eyes.

FIGURE 3-8: Aspartame female with an apparent tumor of the lymph or mammary gland and bleeding eyes.

For a discussion of aspartame and bleeding eyes, see "Bleeding eyes" on page 49.

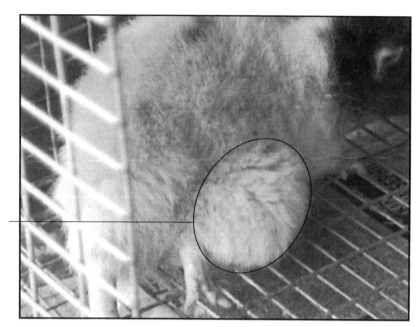

This female appeared to have a lymph or mammary gland tumor in front of her right hind leg.

FIGURE 3-9: Female on aspartame with an apparent lymph or mammary gland tumor.

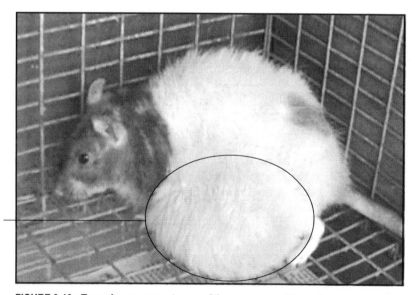

This female had an apparent tumor of the lymph or mammary gland on her left side.

FIGURE 3-10: Female on aspartame with an apparent lymph or mammary gland tumor.

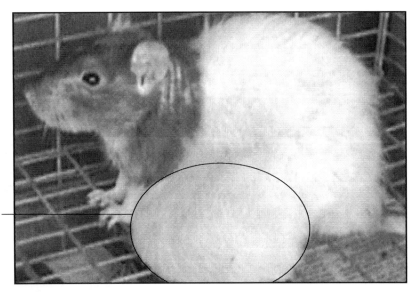

This female had an
apparent tumor of the
lymph or mammary
gland on her
left side.

FIGURE 3-11: Female on aspartame with an apparent lymph or mammary gland tumor.

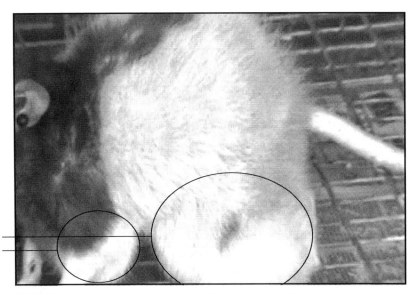

This female had
multiple tumors of the
lymph or mammary
gland on her
left side.

FIGURE 3-12: Female on aspartame with an apparent lymph or mammary gland tumor.

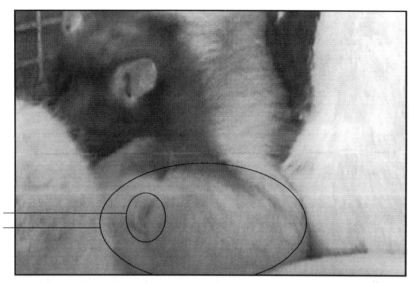

This female developed an apparent lymph or mammary gland tumor that almost completely engulfed her left foreleg.

FIGURE 3-13: Female on aspartame with an apparent lymph or mammary gland tumor.

The female in Figure 3-14 appears to have a tumor of the lymph gland on the left side of her neck.

She also had protruding eyes, a symptom in humans of the thyroid disorder called Grave's disease (see "Protruding eyes" on page 51).

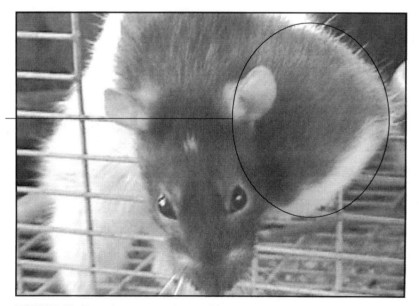

This female appeared to have a lymph gland tumor on the left side of her neck.

FIGURE 3-14: Female on aspartame with an apparent lymph gland tumor and protruding eyes.

Black and brown females with lymph or mammary gland tumors

In my experiment, the brown and black females on aspartame shown in Figure 3-15 through Figure 3-19 had apparent lymph or mammary gland tumors.

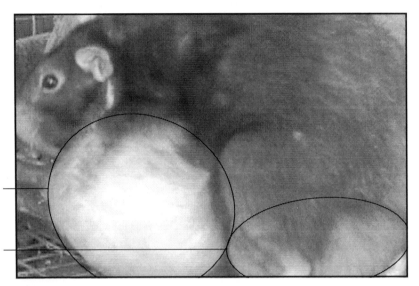

This female developed an apparent lymph gland tumor and a secondary lymph or mammary gland tumor.

FIGURE 3-15: Female on aspartame with an apparent lymph or mammary gland tumor.

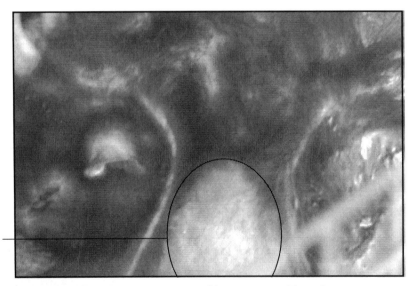

This female appeared to have a lymph or mammary gland tumor behind her left foreleg. She also had thinning fur and skin problems.

FIGURE 3-16: Female on aspartame with an apparent lymph or mammary gland tumor.

The female in Figure 3-16 also had thinning fur and developed severe skin problems as shown in Figure 4-18 (see "Thinning fur" on page 56 and "Skin disorders within my aspartame group" on page 53).

This female appeared to have a lymph or mammary gland tumor on her right side.

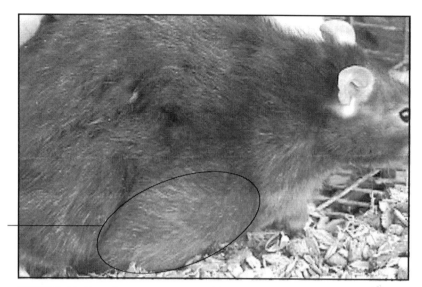

FIGURE 3-17: Female on aspartame with an apparent lymph or mammary gland tumor.

This female appeared to have a lymph or mammary gland tumor on her left side.

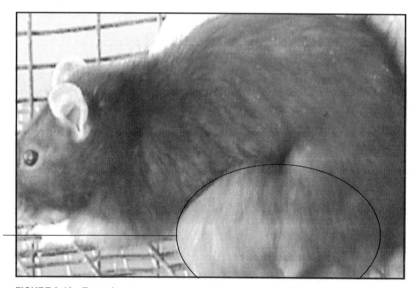

FIGURE 3-18: Female on aspartame with an apparent lymph or mammary gland tumor.

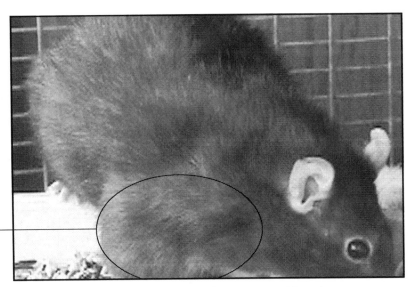

This female appeared to have a lymph or mammary gland tumor behind her right foreleg.

FIGURE 3-19: Female on aspartame with an apparent lymph or mammary gland tumor.

Beige female with lymph or mammary gland tumors

In my experiment, the beige female on aspartame shown in Figure 3-20 developed multiple lymph or mammary gland tumors.

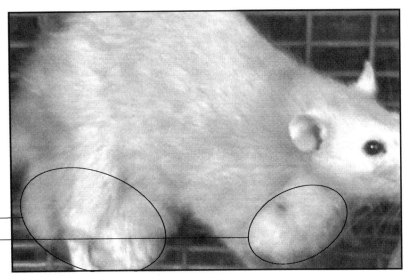

This female appeared to have multiple lymph or mammary gland tumors.

FIGURE 3-20: Female on aspartame with multiple lymph or mammary gland tumors.

Males on aspartame with tumors

The males on aspartame shown in Figure 3-21 through Figure 3-27 had apparent mammary or lymph gland tumors.

Those in Figure 3-21 and Figure 3-23 also appeared to have tinges of yellowing fur, a possible symptom of aspartame poisoning (see "Yellowing fur" on page 58).

This male had a growth on his belly that was possibly a mammary or lymph gland tumor. It made it difficult for him to maintain an upright position.

He also had yellowing fur, a possible symptom of aspartame poisoning.

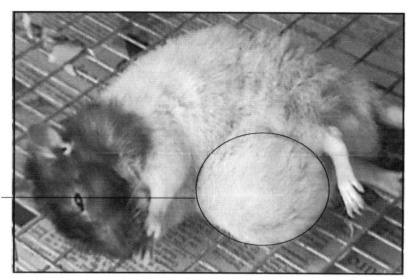

FIGURE 3-21: Male on aspartame with an apparent mammary or lymph gland tumor near his left hind leg.

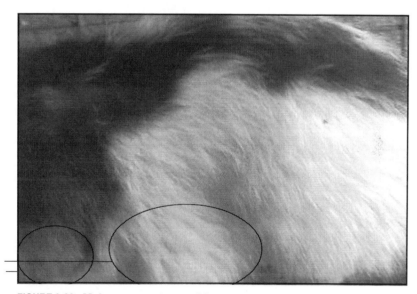

This male had multiple growths near his left foreleg which were apparent mammary or lymph gland tumors.

FIGURE 3-22: Male on aspartame with an apparent lymph gland tumor in front of and mammary or lymph gland tumor behind his left foreleg.

This male had a growth near his right hind leg that appears to have been a mammary or lymph gland tumor.

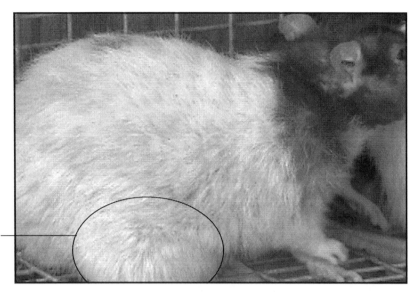

FIGURE 3-23: **Male on aspartame with an apparent mammary or lymph gland tumor above his right hind leg.**

This male had a growth near his right foreleg that appears to have been a mammary or lymph gland tumor.

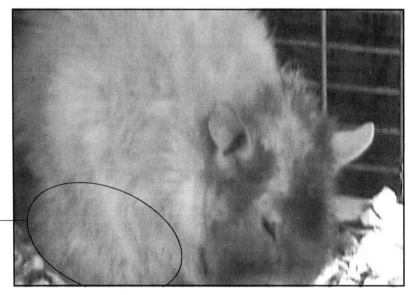

FIGURE 3-24: **Male on aspartame with an apparent mammary or lymph gland tumor near his right foreleg.**

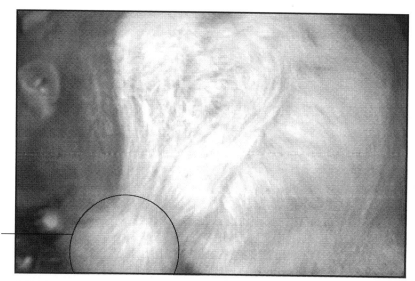

This male had a growth near his left foreleg which appears to have been a mammary or lymph gland tumor.

FIGURE 3-25: Male on aspartame with an apparent mammary or lymph gland tumor near his left foreleg.

The male in Figure 3-25 also grew obese (see "Obesity within my aspartame group" on page 59).

The male in Figure 3-26 had a growth on the left side of his face, which diminished in size after he got into a fight. For more about aspartame and aggressive behavior, see the discussion on page 48.

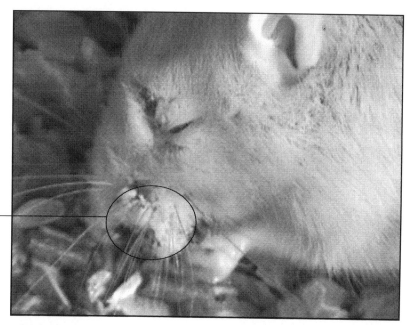

This male had a growth on the left side of his face.

FIGURE 3-26: Male on aspartame who developed a tumor on the left side of his face.

The male on aspartame shown post mortem in Figure 3-27, had a tumor on the right side of his face. I found him a few days after he died hidden behind one of the clay houses in his cage.

This male had a growth on the right side of his face. He was one of the first casualties of my experiment. He died within weeks after it started.

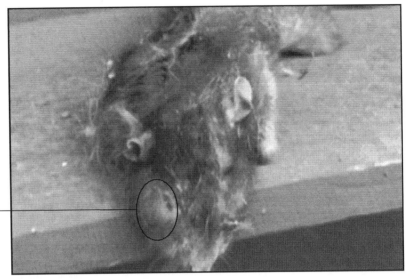

FIGURE 3-27: Male on aspartame who developed a tumor on the right side of his face.

Tumors in my control group

In my experiment, the control females shown in Figure 3-28 through Figure 3-31 developed apparent lymph or mammary gland tumors.

This control female developed an apparent lymph or mammary gland tumor on her left side.

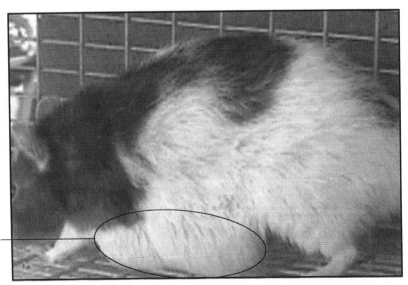

FIGURE 3-28: Female from the control group with an apparent lymph or mammary gland tumor.

This control female developed an apparent lymph or mammary gland tumor near her left foreleg.

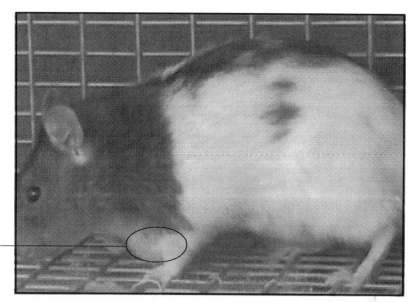

FIGURE 3-29: Control group female with apparent lymph or mammary gland tumor.

This control female developed multiple lymph or mammary gland tumors on her left side.

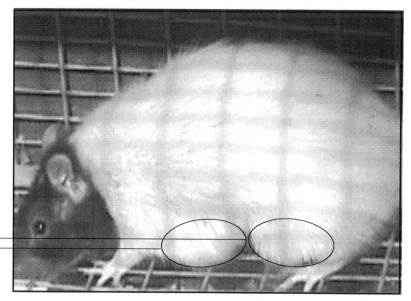

FIGURE 3-30: Control group female with multiple lymph or mammary gland tumors.

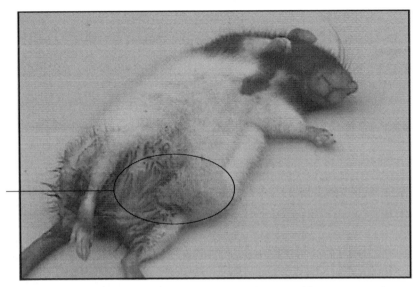

This control female
developed an
apparent lymph or
mammary gland tumor
on her left side.

FIGURE 3-31: White and black control group female with an apparent lymph or mammary gland tumor.

The brown female shown in Figure 3-32 developed an apparent lymph or mammary gland tumor under her right foreleg.

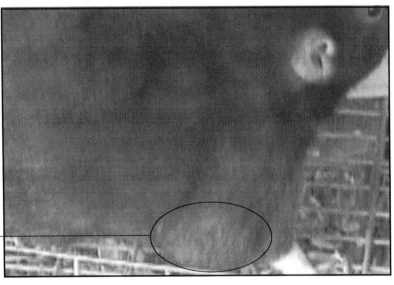

This control female
developed an
apparent lymph or
mammary gland
tumor behind
her right foreleg.

FIGURE 3-32: Brown control group female with an apparent lymph or mammary gland tumor.

For a summary of the results shown in this chapter, see "Conclusion" on page 61.

4   Other Adverse Results

"Let's just have a quick review of what MSG and the excitotoxins [such as aspartame] do. Well, they are associated with neurodegenerative diseases, they are associated with neurodevelopmental abnormalities, nervous system injury ... endocrine disorders, diabetes Types 1 and 2, Syndrome X, gross obesity, enhanced cancer growth and spread, immune dysfunction, retinal disorder, arterial sclerosis, multiple sclerosis, lupus and other auto-immune disorders, GI disorders and sudden cardiac death."[1]

—Dr. Russell Blaylock, neurosurgeon

The above quote exposes the wide range of adverse effects that may be associated with aspartame, now rebranded as AminoSweet.[2] The tumors I observed are shown in Chapter 3. The following subsections show the diversity of additional adverse effects I observed:

- "Neurological disorders within my aspartame group" on page 41
- "Eye disorders within my aspartame group" on page 46
- "Skin disorders within my aspartame group" on page 53
- "Thinning & yellowing fur within my aspartame group" on page 56
- "Obesity within my aspartame group" on page 59

Neurological disorders within my aspartame group

Does aspartame cause neurological disorders? In the Index of *Aspartame Disease, an Ignored Epidemic*, Dr. Roberts lists the following "neurologic complications" that he observed in his patients as possibly being associated with aspartame consumption:

"Alzheimer's, amyotrophic lateral sclerosis (ALS), attention-deficit disorder and hyperactivity, carpal tunnel syndrome, cataplexy, confusion, dizziness, dopa-responsive dystonia, facial pain, hypnagogic hallucinations, intellectual deterioration, memory loss, motor neuron disease, muscle weakness, myasthenia gravis, neuralgia, Parkinson's disease, peripheral neuropathy, pseudotumor cerebri, restless legs syndrome, Sjogren's syndrome, sleep apnea, sleep paralysis, slurring of speech, multiple sclerosis, Tourette's syndrome, tremors, unexplained blackouts, unexplained pain, unsteadiness."[3]

The following subsections show images of my rats on aspartame with visible symptoms of various types of neurological disorders.

Paralysis

"I have been seeing doctors for over three years now trying to find out why I am being turned into a cripple. I have severe weakness in upper legs and upper arms, they have tested me for everything under the sun and keep telling me I do not have anything they recognize.... I started to notice that my bad cycles coincided with how much diet soft drink I was using at the time."[4]

During my experiment, the hind legs of the male on aspartame shown in Figure 4-1 became paralyzed.

The hind legs of this male on aspartame became paralyzed.

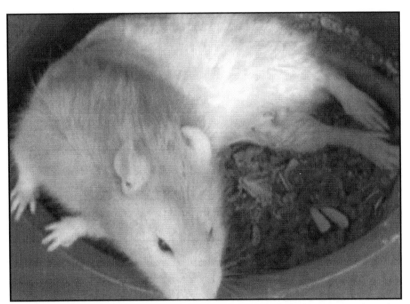

FIGURE 4-1: The hind legs of this male on aspartame became paralyzed

ALS, also known as Lou Gehrig's disease, can lead to paralysis. According to Dr. Blaylock, *"There is growing evidence that excitotoxins* [such as aspartame] *play a major role in a whole group of degenerative brain diseases in adults—especially the elderly. These diseases include Parkinson's disease, Alzheimer's disease, Huntington's disease.... ALS, as well as several more rare disorders of the nervous system."*[5]

Spasmodic torticollis

Figure 4-2 shows a female on aspartame who continually twisted her head to her left, similar to the human disease, idiopathic spasmodic torticollis[6] (IST). eMedicine states that: *"Torticollis is a condition that causes the neck to involuntarily twist to one side secondary to contraction of the neck muscles. The ear is tilted toward the contracted muscle and the chin is facing the opposite direction."* It is interesting to note that eMedicine states that torticollis may be chemically induced.[7]

The neck of this female on aspartame was continually twisted to the left.

In humans, this is a symptom of the neurological disorder spasmodic torticollis, also referred to as dystonia.

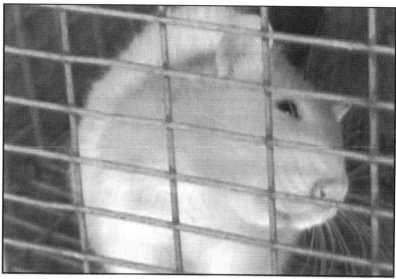

FIGURE 4-2: This female on aspartame appeared to have torticollis

In *Aspartame Disease, an Ignored Epidemic*, H.J. Roberts, MD, discusses dopa-responsive dystonia as being affected by the ingestion of aspartame because of its breakdown component phenylalanine: "*Hereditary progressive dystonia is another neurologic disorder that usually affects children.... Patients with this condition (at times misdiagnosed as cerebral palsy) can be adversely affected by ingesting phenylalanine because of decreased hepatic phenylalanine hydroxylase activity.*"[8]

Cerebral palsy

"*During my pregnancy with my nine year old, I consumed sugar-free frozen yogurt (I craved it!) and he was born four months early, weighed one pound, nine ounces and now suffers from cerebral palsy and mental retardation. Until now, we all assumed that these were both due solely to premature birth. Now I wonder if he was born prematurely because I consumed aspartame and if so, did the aspartame cause all of this?*"[9]

I was unable to capture it on camera, but one of my females continually moved her head from side to side, a possible symptom of cerebral palsy.[10]

According to aspartame investigator and victim Jim Bowen, MD, and former FDA investigator Arthur M. Evangelista, "*During maternal aspartame consumption, development of the fetal nervous system is damaged or impaired via excitotoxic-saturated placental blood flow that can cause or contribute to cerebral palsy and pervasive developmental disorders....*

"*This is due to an incompetent blood brain barrier and neuronal (brain) damage produced by excitotoxins circulating in the fetal brain areas. This is especially true for those areas adjacent to the brain's ventricular system. There is no doubt that destruction or damage to the hypothalamus and corresponding neuro-endocrine organs leads to potential developmental complications (physical and mental).*"[11]

Dr. Louis Elsas, then director of Emory University School of Medicine, Department of Pediatrics, Division of Medical Genetics, testified before Congress on November 3, 1987, that he had spent 25 years *"trying to prevent mental retardation and birth defects caused by excess phenylalanine. And herein lies my basic concern, that aspartame is in fact a well known neurotoxin and teratogen which, in some as yet undefined dose, will both reversibly in the adult and irreversibly in the developing child or fetal brain, produce adverse effects."*[12]

"Many studies of both acute and chronic ingestion of 34 mg aspartame/kg/day have demonstrated a two- to five-fold increase in semi-fasting blood phenylalanine concentrations (from approximately 50 to 250 μM) without concomitant increases in tyrosine or other amino acids. The degree of increase by normal humans depends on several variables including the efficiency of gut transport, liver utilization and growth rates. It was thought by many scientists that this degree of blood phenylalanine increase would not affect brain function. However, currently available information indicates that this is not true.

"In the developing fetus such a rise in maternal blood phenylalanine could be magnified four to six fold by the concentrative efforts of the placenta and fetal blood brain barrier. Thus, a maternal phenylalanine of 150 μM could reach 900 μM in the developing fetal brain cell and this concentration kills such cells in tissue culture. The effect of such an increased fetal brain concentration in vivo would probably be much more subtle and expressed as mental retardation, microcephaly, or potentially certain birth defects.

"In the rapidly growing post-natal brain (children of 0-12 months) irreversible brain damage could occur by the same mechanism.

"In the adult, we have found that changes in blood phenylalanine in these concentration ranges are associated with slowing of the electroencephalogram, and prolongation of cognitive function tests. Fortunately, these effects on the mature brain are reversible but provide clear evidence for a negative effect on sensitive parameters of brain function."[13]

Difficulty walking

"The top of my feet have become numb and my walking gait has changed.... The only aspartame that I consume is from sugarless gum. I had been chewing up to 24 pieces per day. Is that enough to cause problems?"

"I am a 68 year old male. I have been a runner and then a walker for the last 26 years, until I developed a problem with my feet. The top of my feet have become numb and my walking gait has changed. I went to the doc, he did a brain and back scan. The results came back OK. I would walk 10 to 12 miles per day at a 14 minute pace, 6 days a week.... Since my walking gait has changed, my pace has slowed and I am not as steady as I had been.... On the web, I found a connection with walking gait change, foot drop and MS [multi-

ple sclerosis]. *The only aspartame that I consume is from sugarless gum. I had been chewing up to 24 pieces per day. Is that enough to cause problems?"*[14]

> ***Note: According to the website aspartamekills.com, "In the May 1992 edition of their journal, Flying Safety, the United States Air Force warned all pilots to stay off aspartame, stating: 'Some people have suffered aspartame related disorders with doses as small as that carried in a single stick of chewing gum.'"***[15]
>
> ***According to Jim Bowen, MD, "Aspartame in chewing gum is absorbed directly though the buccal mucosa of the tongue, mouth, and gums, making it a far worse poisoning than even if it were given intravenously. The nerves serving this area and their vascular supply derive directly from the brain, so the aspartame absorbed through them goes directly into the brain, by-passing the spinal cord and blood brain barrier."***[16]

The male on aspartame shown in Figure 4-3 had trouble walking and frequently fell over. His body leaned toward the left. He also appeared to have mild symptoms of torticollis. See "Spasmodic torticollis" on page 42.

While walking, this male on aspartame continually leaned toward his left.

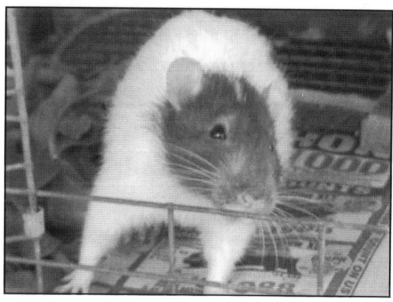

FIGURE 4-3: Male on aspartame with difficulty walking and mild symptoms of torticollis

The female on aspartame shown in Figure 4-4 also had trouble walking.

This female on aspartame also leaned toward her left as she walked.

Her leaning is so extreme in this photo, it looks as if she is falling.

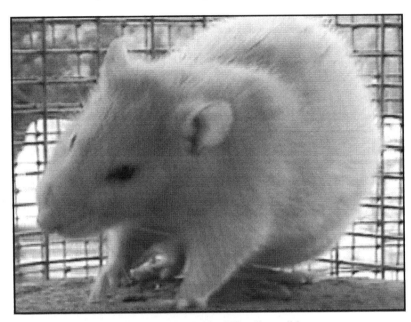

FIGURE 4-4: Female on aspartame with difficulty walking

Eye disorders within my aspartame group

"For many years I had consumed four to five diet sodas daily. I am a jogger and very active with a pretty good diet.... In 2002 I had an eye infection and had to see an ophthalmologist who told me I had a fairly advanced cataract in one eye and the beginnings in the other. My father had them so I assumed that this was genetics. In August, 2004 I went back for a check-up and the ophthalmologist said that he felt that I should consider surgery on the left eye. I put it off. Then I received some of the material about aspartame from a friend.... As I read this stuff I could not believe how many of the symptoms they described fit me. After quitting aspartame for approximately two months I had my most recent eye exam in Aug. 05. The quote: 'Your eyes look fantastic.... no surgery needed.'"[17]

The following subsections shows rats on aspartame with eye infections, bleeding, and protruding eyes.

Eye infections

According to Dr. Janet Starr Hull, when consuming aspartame you are more likely to have an increased susceptibility to infection.[18] Dr. Roberts reports possible correlations between aspartame consumption and infection, including that associated with acquired immune deficiency syndrome (AIDS), chronic Epstein-Barr infection, rheumatic fever, and yeast infection.[19]

Regarding the possible mechanisms involved, Dr. Roberts states that:

"Increased phenylalanine [a breakdown component of aspartame] *appears to alter cell-mediated immunity. This is evidenced by the enhanced immunity*

noted in both animals and humans placed on phenylalanine restriction. In turn, elevation of the serum phenylalanine by infection can contribute to a vicious cycle. The phenylalanine/large neutral amino acid ratio increases in acute infection by as much as 50 percent.[20] "

I observed two males and a female on aspartame with eye infections, as shown in Figure 4-5 through Figure 4-7.

This male and the female below developed eye infections.

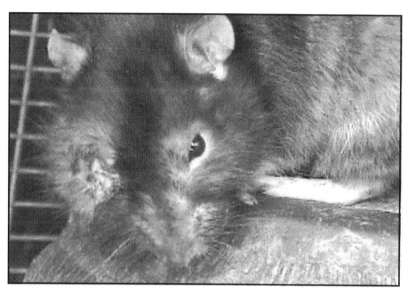

FIGURE 4-5: Male on aspartame with an infection in his right eye

The eyes of the female on aspartame in Figure 4-6 also became infected.

Note the eye puffiness and pool of blood under her left eye.

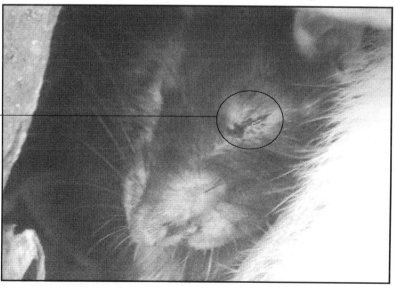

FIGURE 4-6: Female on aspartame with infected eyes

The female in Figure 4-6 also had bleeding eyes, a possible symptom of aspartame poisoning. See "Bleeding eyes" on page 49.

The male in Figure 4-7 developed an eye infection after a fight.

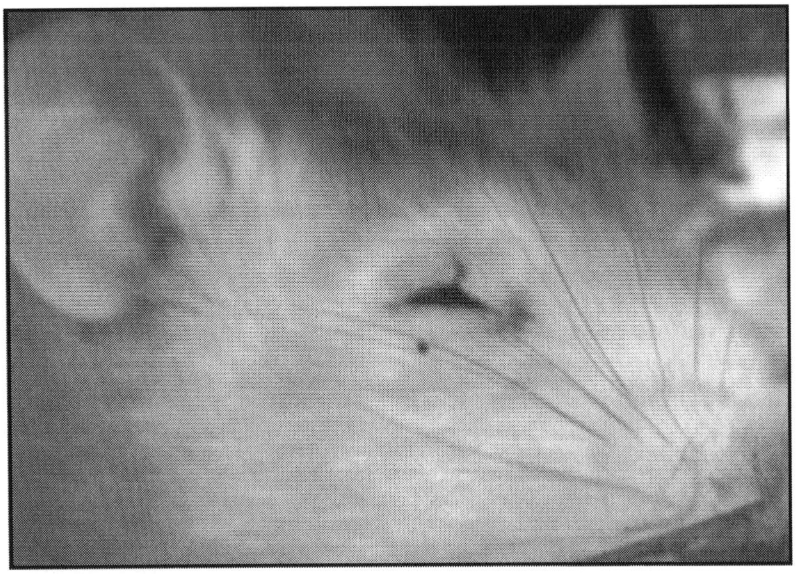

FIGURE 4-7: This male on aspartame also had an eye infection

> **The rats on aspartame seemed significantly more aggressive than the controls.**

Speaking of fighting, the rats on aspartame seemed significantly more aggressive than the controls. I once saw two males on aspartame on their hind legs fighting violently. The controls were relatively passive. According to the *National PKU News*, a high blood level of phenylalanine, the majority breakdown (50%) component of aspartame, may induce aggressive behavior in people with phenylketonuria (PKU), an inborn disorder of phenylalanine metabolism often associated with mental retardation in children.[22] The tendency toward aggressive behavior is elucidated by a concerned teen in the Q&A section of the *National PKU News*:

"Q. Is there a relationship between PKU and aggressive tendencies? I am a teen who has a problem with becoming extremely angry and aggressive, almost violent at times. Is this common, or is it just me?

"A. This behavior suggests to me that you are either off the [PKU] diet, or if you are on the diet that your blood phe [phenylalanine] levels are too high. PKU patients who are off diet or whose levels are too high are often aggressive and less stable."[23]

Several studies cited in an article entitled "Behavioral and Neurological Effects of Aspartame," claim that a diet excessive in phenylalanine *can induce PKU*,[24] and can therefore induce aggressive behavior. Such behavior may be explained by how phenylalanine is processed by the blood-brain barrier before entering the brain. When ingested, digested, and carried to the blood-brain barrier, phenylalanine competes with the amino acid tyrosine to become attached to the neutral amino acid that transports it to the brain.[25] When excess phenylalanine is consumed, the brain gets less tyrosine, found in high concentrations in meats, whole grains, dairy, avocados, bananas, legumes, beans and nuts.[26] After entering the brain, tyrosine is converted into norepinephrine and dopamine.[27] Norepinephrine is a mood elevator that stimulates a sense of well being,[28] and its depletion can lead to depression, which can in turn, lead to aggression. In a study of 42 normal women and 23 normal men, aggression and depression were found to have a significant positive correlation for the women, but not the men.[29] A study of 1101 persons with dementia found those manifesting physical or verbal aggression had a higher prevalence of depression.[30] When 2083 Norwegian pupils in Grade 8 were surveyed, a significant positive correlation was found between depression and aggressive, bullying behavior.[31] An analysis of surveys taken for 41 eleven-year-olds and 22 fifteen-year-olds found significant correlations between depression and aggression in the 11-year-olds, and an even stronger correlation among the 15-year-olds.[32]

> *Note: The depletion of dopamine due to the over-consumption of phenylalanine can lead to Parkinson's disease. Several drugs are sold to treat the disease by increasing dopamine levels in the brain.[33] Dr. Blaylock began a 20-year quest for the causes of Parkinson's after his father died from it in March, 1989. Blaylock found that Parkinson's, Alzheimer's, and Lou Gehrig's diseases may be correlated with the use of aspartame, MSG, and other neurotoxic chemicals he discusses in Excitotoxins: the Taste that Kills.[34]*

The saturation of phenylalanine from aspartame consumption can also lead to the depletion of the amino acid tryptophan, a precursor of serotonin,[35] thought to be involved in the control of appetite, sleep, memory, learning, temperature, mood, behavior (including sexual and hallucinogenic), the cardiovascular system, muscle contractions, the endocrine system, and depression.[36]

When aspartame is consumed over time, the resulting depletion of tryptophan can cause depression and aggressive behavior due to a lack of serotonin in the brain and spinal fluid.

Phenylalanine, tyrosine, and tryptophan are classified by biochemists as aromatic amino acids because of their chemical structures. As such, they compete with one another to pass through the blood-brain barrier.[37] When aspartame is consumed over time, the resulting depletion of tryptophan can cause depression and aggressive behavior due to a lack of serotonin in the brain and spinal fluid.[38] Three studies done by the University of Texas using 24 men, 8 men, and 12 women, respectively, found that when subjects were provoked, aggressive incidents increased under tryptophan-depleted conditions and decreased when blood levels of tryptophan were elevated.[39, 40, 41]

Six other studies have correlated serotonin depletion with impulsive and violent criminal behaviors. Six more have associated the condition with alcohol abuse and dependence. Three studies have correlated a lack of serotonin with Gilles de la Tourette's syndrome. Two studies associated a lack of serotonin with bulimia. Four studies have associated serotonin depletion with suicide attempts, and three have associated it with children institutionalized for aggressive behavior.[42]

Bleeding eyes

In addition to bleeding in the eyes of the female in Figure 4-6, the eyes of the male on aspartame shown in Figure 4-8 were visibly bleeding.

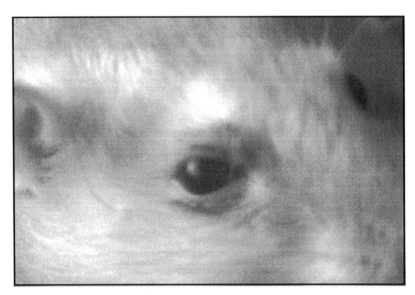

FIGURE 4-8: This male on aspartame had bleeding eyes

The eyes in the female on aspartame shown in Figure 4-9 were infected and bleeding. This female also had a mammary or lymph gland tumor as shown in Figure 3-8.

The eyes in the female on aspartame shown in Figure 4-9 were infected and bleeding.

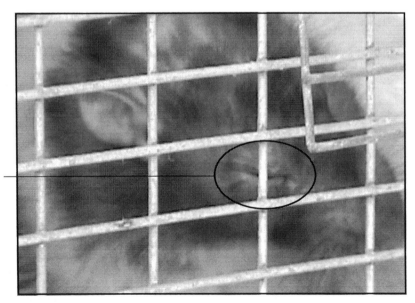

Bleeding eye ———

FIGURE 4-9: This female on aspartame had bleeding eyes

Bleeding eyes have also been found to occur in humans consuming aspartame. According to psychiatrist Ralph Walton, MD, *"In our double-blind study here at this hospital, we had a really tragic situation which occurred, which I attributed directly to the aspartame. We needed volunteers. We looked at both patients, that is people who had a history of a mood disorder. And we needed some controls, that is, people without a history of mood disorder.*

One of the people that I used [in the aspartame group of] *the study was the administrator for our psychiatric staff with a PhD in psychology. Several days into the study he had sudden bleeding in his eye and a detachment of his retina, and had to be rushed to Cleveland for emergency surgery. His eye could not be saved. He lost the vision in one eye. At the same time, we had another participant in* [the aspartame group of] *this study—a nurse—who also had bleeding in her eye. So we had two people who during the course of the study had eye emergencies."*[43] Dr. Walton subsequently discontinued the study.

Protruding eyes

The female on aspartame shown in Figure 4-10 had protruding eyes—a symptom of the thyroid disorder called Grave's disease in humans.[44]

According to Dr. Janet Starr Hull, *"In 1991, I was diagnosed with an 'incurable' case of Grave's Disease, a fatal thyroid disorder. I never really had Grave's Disease but my doctors were convinced I did. I had aspartame poisoning with symptoms of 'textbook' Grave's Disease caused by aspartame saturating my foods."*[45]

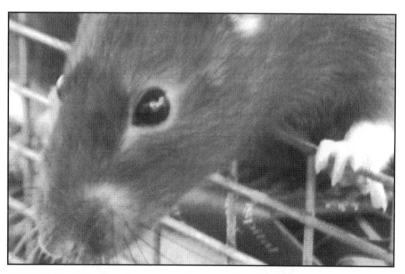

FIGURE 4-10: This female on aspartame had protruding eyes

Dr. Hull continues:

I had protruding eyes, cystic acne, and my hair was falling out in clumps. I had gained 30 pounds, too. ALL that went away within a year from stopping all aspartame. I even had holes in my retina from the methanol,[1] and those have closed up now. All backed up by my eye surgeon."[46]

---

1. Methanol is a breakdown component of aspartame.

The females on aspartame shown in Figure 4-11 and Figure 4-12 also had protruding eyes.

Protruding eyes are a symptom of the thyroid disorder called Grave's Disease

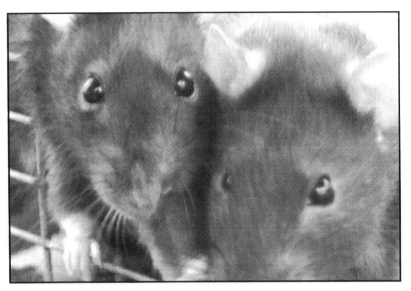

FIGURE 4-11: Females on aspartame with protruding eyes

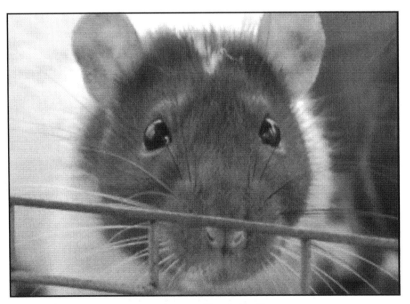

FIGURE 4-12: Female on aspartame with protruding eyes

Blindness

"Several years ago I used to consume about one roll of aspartame-containing mints per day. After having an eye exam where the doctor performed the 'air jet' test, I developed obliterative vasculitis. The tiny veins in my eyes were breaking and bleeding, which nearly blinded my left eye."

"Several years ago I used to consume about one roll of aspartame-containing mints per day. After having an eye exam where the doctor performed the 'air jet' test, I developed obliterative vasculitis. The tiny veins in my eyes were breaking and bleeding, which nearly blinded my left eye. (I quit those mints MANY years ago but should have done so sooner). I then went to another eye doctor who performed laser eye surgery and completely healed my right eye. The left eye was mostly healed, but now I suffer from macular degeneration or warping in that eye. It is like having a movable black zone or blind spot, but fortunately my right eye has been able to compensate. The vision tester at the DMV thought I was completely blind in that eye."[47]

I was unable to get video, and it probably would have been difficult to see in a photo, but one of my females on aspartame acted as if she were blind. Blindness has also been reported as one of the adverse effects of methanol, a breakdown component of aspartame.

Skin disorders within my aspartame group

By 1987 the FDA had already received over 3,600 consumer complaints about aspartame.[48] The Aspartame Consumer Safety Network reported in 1996 that they had filed over 10,000 consumer complaints with the FDA.[49] The adverse effects attributed to aspartame in complaints submitted to the FDA were published in April 1995 by the FDA's parent organization, the Department of Health and Human Services (HHS). The data was obtained by a Freedom of Information Act (FOIA) request by reporter Barbara Mullarkey.[50] It included a list of 92 symptoms reportedly resulting from aspartame[51] that shows 114 people reporting skin problems.

Figure 4-13 shows an open ulcer that never healed, found above the right hind leg of a male on aspartame.

Open ulcer on a male on aspartame.

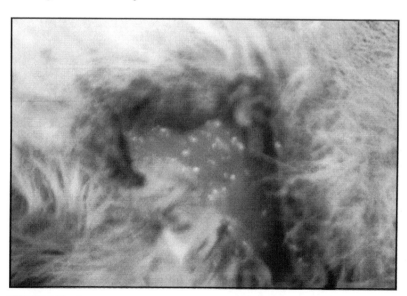

FIGURE 4-13: Open ulcer that never healed on a male on aspartame

These males on aspartame developed skin lesions.

The males on aspartame in Figure 4-14 through Figure 4-17 had skin lesions.

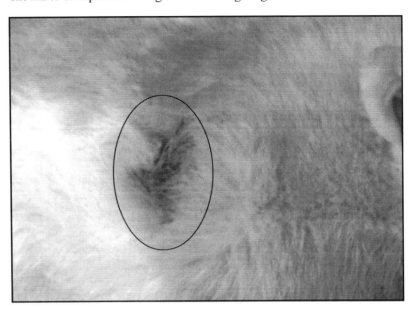

FIGURE 4-14: Male on aspartame with a skin lesion

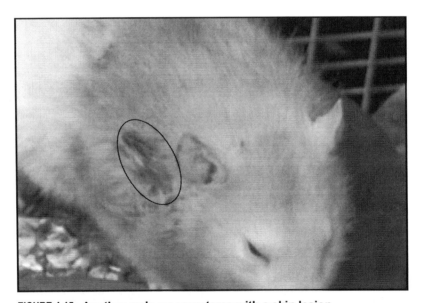

FIGURE 4-15: Another male on aspartame with a skin lesion

These males on aspartame also developed skin lesions.

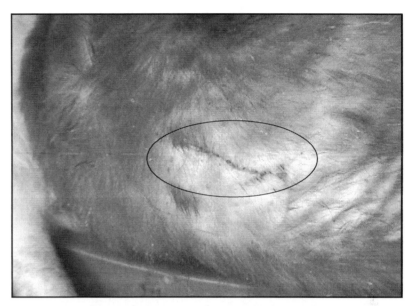

FIGURE 4-16: Another male on aspartame with a skin lesion

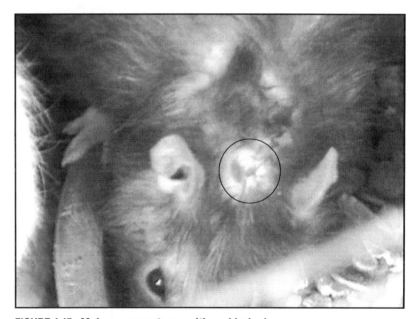

FIGURE 4-17: Male on aspartame with a skin lesion

The male in Figure 4-17 had a skin lesion and thinning fur. Also see "Thinning fur" on page 56.

About one-third of the skin on the back of the aspartame female shown in Figure 4-18 became separated from her body about a week before she died.

The skin of this female started coming off a week before she died.

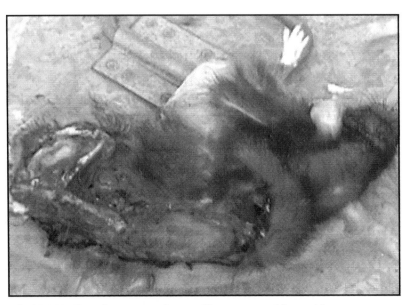

FIGURE 4-18: Female on aspartame with a severe skin problem

Thinning & yellowing fur within my aspartame group

The following subsections describe rats with thinning and yellowing fur.

Thinning fur

"I was buying 12 packs of Diet Coke.... I would grab a 12 pack every other day.... On March 11th, 1999 ... I was feeling very sick. I hadn't felt good for a few years now. I was always tired. Full of aches and pains. Felt like I was ready to have my 90th birthday. That is when I realized how much Diet Coke had taken over my life. So what symptoms did I have? ... Thirst - Weight gain (50 lb.) - Tired all the time - Aches in my joints - Throbbing headaches - Hair loss - Blurred vision - Mood swings - Depression - Couldn't think straight - Lived in a haze - Cramps - Rashes - Numbness in my legs & arms - Confusion....

"My mother ... was worried about my consumption of Diet Coke.... Mother had heard about ... how aspartame was bad for you and caused brain cancer. Well ... I shrugged it off.

"By the time I figured out what was causing it, I had lost about half my hair volume."

"The hair loss caused me great pain. As a teenager I had the thickest most beautiful hair. I would comb my hair and have a sink full of it. Just running my hands through my hair would produce a handful. It fell out all over the place.... By the time I figured out what was causing it, I had lost about half my hair volume.

"On March 11th, 1999 ... I was talking to my boyfriend and for some reason I picked up my Diet Coke can. The word ASPARTAME stuck out at me.... So I

typed in aspartame into Excite and I found www.aspartamekills.com.... I dumped my Diet Coke out and I have not touched it since.

"All those symptoms above I listed. They are all gone. Every one of them. My hair is even growing back. I can comb my hair without a ton of hair on my brush instead of my head. My hair stopped falling out within a week. It is amazing how I feel."[52]

The males on aspartame shown in Figure 4-19 and Figure 4-20 had thinning fur.

"All those symptoms above I listed. They are all gone. Every one of them. My hair is even growing back. I can comb my hair without a ton of hair on my brush instead of my head. My hair stopped falling out within a week. It is amazing how I feel."

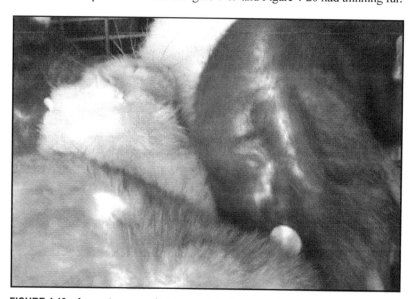

FIGURE 4-19: Aspartame males started losing their fur.

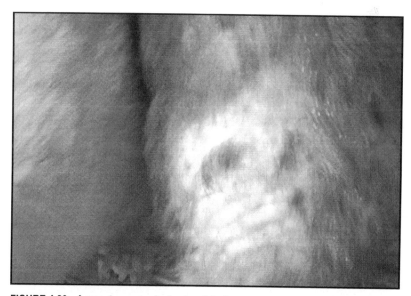

FIGURE 4-20: Aspartame male losing his fur.

A few of the rats in the control group also developed thinning fur, so I thought it may be part of the normal aging process. However, some suspect that aspartame is the cause of their hair loss. Recall that Dr. Janet Hull complained of "*hair falling out in clumps*" in the quote on page 51, and here's another person's experience:

"I am a 40 year old woman.... Until six months ago I had glorious, thick auburn hair. Now, I have the horseshoe patterns with tufts of hair on top, as is frequently seen in balding men.

"I have always consumed 3 to 6 diet sodas per day, and have never noticed any problems with my hair until recently.... About a year ago I decided to make a conscious effort to eliminate all refined sugar and high fructose corn syrup from my diet. This eliminated not just any candy, cookies, ice cream, etc., but also most fruit juices (read the labels!) and also, fruit flavored yogurt and fruit preserves/jams/jellies. I replaced these items in my diet with 'Lite' versions, which contain NutraSweet (aspartame)....

> *"[My] hair started falling out in clumps and within the passing of two months, I had lost more than half of the hair on my head!"*

"For a few months, I noticed that my scalp felt 'tight.' ... Then, the hair started falling out in clumps and within the passing of two months, I had lost more than half of the hair on my head! My scalp is now clearly visible over the top and sides of my head, and the hair in the back of my head is noticeably (to me) thinner.

Any time I touch my head, my hand comes away with 10 or more hairs, which are very thin at the scalp end (the recent growth of 1/4 inch is less than half the thickness of the rest of the strand) and the root is still attached when the hair falls out. Does anyone else suspect their alopecia is due to use of NutraSweet?!?!?!?[53]

Yellowing fur

According to the book *The Rat*,[54] yellowing fur can be an effect of the natural aging process. The World Health Organization, however, reports that yellowing fur can be a symptom of formaldehyde exposure.[55] Formaldehyde is a breakdown component of the methyl-alcohol component of aspartame. Formaldehyde has been shown to collect and persist in vital organs after the consumption of aspartame. According to the Trocho study:

"The chronic treatment of a series of rats with 200 mg/kg of non-labelled [non-radioactive] *aspartame during 10 days resulted in the accumulation of even more label* [radioactive formaldehyde] *when given the radioactive bolus* [a very large amount of radioactive aspartame administered at a single time], *suggesting that the amount of formaldehyde adducts* [the accumulation of formaldehyde bound to proteins] *coming from aspartame in tissue proteins and nucleic acids may be cumulative. It is concluded that aspar-*

tame consumption may constitute a hazard because of its contribution to the formation of formaldehyde adducts."[56]

> *Note: My understanding of this quote is that when the body is still metabolizing non-radioactive formaldehyde that has accumulated from previous doses, and is then given a large amount of radioactive aspartame at a single time (a bolus), then more of the radioactive formaldehyde accumulates in the body because the non-radioactive formaldehyde is still being metabolized.*

Formaldehyde adducts are difficult to eliminate from the body. They damage the nervous and immune systems and cause irreversible genetic damage.[57]

Formaldehyde is often found in dark wines.[58] A few years ago, a friend became the caregiver for her 80-something year-old father who had been given copious amounts of wine by his previous caregiver, and his hair had yellowed. When he stopped drinking the wine, the yellowing disappeared.

In my experiment, the females on aspartame shown in Figure 3-4 through Figure 3-13 and the males on aspartame shown in Figure 3-21 and Figure 3-22, appear to have yellow tinges or patches on their otherwise white fur. The white and black control females shown in Figure 3-28 through Figure 3-31 also appeared to have yellowing fur, though in general the yellowing appeared to be significantly less than on the fur of the white and black females in the aspartame group.

> *Note: I was unaware of the issues surrounding yellowing fur until writing this report, and therefore did not look for it on my rats during the experiment. So there may have been others with yellowing fur that I did not photograph. I apologize that the yellowing cannot be seen in the black-and-white version of this report.*

Obesity within my aspartame group

"Consuming aspartame seems to trigger a hunger type feeling, even if I have just eaten, whereas if I abstain from aspartame, I would be satisfied. Does this have any scientific validity, or am I just imagining it? I really get ravenous after consuming 'straight' aspartame like in a diet coke, versus aspartame added to a food, like a milkshake or oatmeal sweetened w/ aspartame."[59]

During my experiment, the female on aspartame in Figure 4-21 grew obese. The male with a tumor shown in Figure 3-25 also grew obese.

This female grew fat.

None of the rats from the control group became fat.

Ironically, aspartame is sold to help people lose weight.

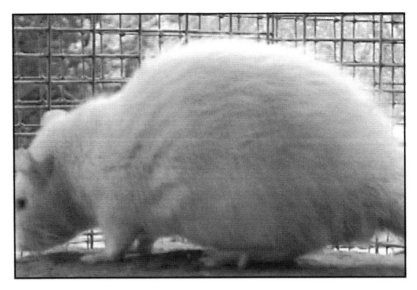

FIGURE 4-21: Female on aspartame that became obese

For more about aspartame, MSG, and obesity, and for my own personal story, see "Does Aspartame Make You Fat?" on page 69.

What could be worse than a diet product that makes you fat? One that is also addictive! See "Is Aspartame Addictive?" on page 75.

Miscellaneous adverse effects in my control group

All rats in my control group were free of visible symptoms of neurological damage. Some males from the control group developed thinning fur. One female from the control group had skin problems.

All rats in my control group were free of visible symptoms of neurological damage. Some males from the group developed thinning fur. One female from the group had skin problems; however, the damage appears to have occurred after death (see Figure 3-31 on page 40). Some females from the control group appeared to have yellowing fur, but not as yellowed as the fur of the rats in the aspartame group. See "Yellowing fur" on page 58.

When a preliminary version of this report was summarized and leaked on the Internet without my permission, it caused a stir on blogs reddit.com and digg.com. See "Misinformation About My Experiment" on page 81. One blogger commented that my control group was too healthy compared to those from other studies. The person claimed that I must have faked my data. See "Did I Fake My Data?" on page 91.

I had actually been concerned when my controls started developing tumors, and investigated possible causes such as pesticides and herbicides in their food. See my frightening findings in "What may have caused my control group tumors?" on page 99. After being accused of falsifying my data, I researched possible reasons my control group may have been healthier than those in other studies. See "Why was my control group relatively healthy?" on page 114.

5 Conclusion

"Prior to the marketing of aspartame, numerous studies were done to evaluate its metabolism and tolerance in healthy subjects and various subpopulations. Postmarketing, numerous additional studies were done, including studies to evaluate alleged sensitivity to aspartame.[1] ... [These studies indicate that aspartame] *does not produce adverse effects, even at doses several orders of magnitude greater than human consumption rates."*[2]

—Dr. Harriett H. Butchko, MD, Director of Clinical Research, Worldwide Regulatory Sciences at Monsanto Company, formerly at The NutraSweet Company; Dr. Frank N. Kotsonis, PhD, Corporate Vice President of Worldwide Regulatory Sciences at Monsanto Company, formerly Sr. Vice President of Preclinical & Clinical Research at The NutraSweet Company, formerly Director of Toxicology at G.D. Searle and Company; Dr. W. Wayne Stargel, Pharm.D., Director of Clinical Research, Worldwide Regulatory Sciences at Monsanto Company and formerly at The NutraSweet Company; Dr. Christian Tschanz, MD, Senior Director of Clinical Research, Worldwide Regulatory Sciences at Monsanto Company and formerly at The NutraSweet Company.

This chapter presents a summary of the data I observed during my aspartame experiment. See these appendices for additional information and analyses:

- "What is Aspartame?" on page 67
- "Does Aspartame Make You Fat?" on page 69
- "Is Aspartame Addictive?" on page 75
- "Misinformation About My Experiment" on page 81
- "What They Say About My Experiment" on page 85
- "Did I Fake My Data?" on page 91
- "For More Info" on page 121

Summary of my experimental results

Out of the 108 rats in my study, 30 males and 30 females—a total of 60 rats—received aspartame (now rebranded as AminoSweet[3]) in the form of NutraSweet mixed in their drinking water. The control group consisted of 24 females and 24 males—a total of 48 rats.

Tumors in my aspartame group

The photos in "Resulting Tumors" starting on page 19 show:

A total of 20 females
from my aspartame
group developed
visible tumors.

That's 20/30 = 2/3 =
67% of all my females
on aspartame.

- A total of 20 females from my aspartame group developed visible tumors (see Figure 3-1 through Figure 3-20). That's 20/30 = 2/3 = 67% of all my females on aspartame.

- Seven males from my aspartame group developed visible tumors (see Figure 3-21 through Figure 3-27). That's 7/30 = 23% of all my males on aspartame.

The total number of rats—both male and female—in my aspartame group with visible tumors was 27/60 = 45%.

Possible reasons for the astronomical number of tumors in my females on aspartame are analyzed in "Why so many tumors in my females on aspartame?" on page 93.

Tumors in my control group

Five females from my control group developed visible tumors (see Figure 3-28 through Figure 3-32). That's 5/24 = 21% of my female controls. No males from my control group developed visible tumors, so the total number of tumors in my control group was 5, or 5/48 = 10%. Tumors in my aspartame group generally grew much larger than those in the control group. Until I learned that most if not all rat experiments result in tumors in their control groups, I was concerned about the tumors within my control group. For a frightening analysis of why my control group females may have developed tumors, see "What may have caused my control group tumors?" on page 99.

Other adverse effects in my aspartame group

In addition to tumors, the rats in my aspartame group developed other health problems, as described in "Other Adverse Results" starting on page 41. These results include:

- Four apparent neurological disorders. See "Neurological disorders within my aspartame group" on page 41.

- Eight apparent eye disorders. See "Eye disorders within my aspartame group" on page 46.

- Six apparent skin disorders. See "Skin disorders within my aspartame group" on page 53.

- Two apparent cases of thinning fur, and 12 apparent cases of yellowing fur. See "Thinning & yellowing fur within my aspartame group" on page 56.

Other adverse effects in my control group

In addition to the tumors shown in the previous chapter, my control group developed other health problems, as described in "Miscellaneous adverse effects in my control group" on page 60.

These results include:

- Three males developed thinning fur.

- One female had skin problems; however, the damage appears to have occurred after death (see Figure 3-31 on page 40).

Did my experiment demonstrate adverse effects of aspartame?

Though I did not have necropsies performed on the rats in my study, I believe that a significant number of the tumors I observed were indeed cancerous.

Though I did not have necropsies performed on the rats in my study, I believe that a significant number of the tumors I observed were indeed cancerous. I also believe that there were cancers that I did not see. I base these opinions on necropsies I had done on rats from a multi-generational aspartame experiment I undertook after completing the experiment documented in this report. I stopped the second experiment midway because it was too difficult to do on my own, it got out of hand, and I realized I could not provide adequate data to justify continuing.

During that experiment, I had three rats on aspartame necropsied by the county veterinarian. (I was unaware of that service during my previous experiment.) Of the rats I had necropsied, one had visible tumors and the others appeared to be in good health before their deaths.

The tumors I observed on one of the rats—a black and white male—did in fact turn out to be cancerous. Malignant tumors were also found in both its armpits and liver that I had not observed.

Here are the diagnoses from the pathologist:

- *"Malignant lymphoma, submandibular* [cancer of the lymph gland under each side of the lower jaw; each with a diameter of 5 cm = 2 in, which I observed] *and axillary lymph nodes* [in each armpit; each with a diameter of 2 cm = 0.8 in, which I did *not* observe.]

- *Fibrosarcoma, skin on top of head* [a malignant tumor of fibrous connective tissue, with a diameter of 2.5 cm = 1 in, which I observed]

- *Hepatoma, focal, liver* [tumor of the liver, with a diameter of 3 mm = 0.12 in, which I did *not* observe]"[4]

The two rats that appeared to be healthy were females. One was found to have malignant tumors. Her pathology report shows these diagnoses:

- *Chondrosarcomas (lung)* [cancerous tumors, each with a diameter of 0.1 - 0.3 cm = 0.03 - 0.1 in]

- *Fibroadenoma (mammary gland)* [cancerous tumor measuring 4 x 2.5 x 2 cm^3 = 1.6 x 1 x 0.8 in^3]

The pathologist made the following comment about this female:

"The large tumor within the lung has formed multiple metastases within the lung itself. The inflammation in the surrounding lung tissue is due to compression and obstruction by the tumors. Evidence of infectious pulmonary diseases (bacterial or viral) is not observed."[5]

No cancer was found in the second rat that appeared healthy. Cause of death was reportedly meningitis. Her kidneys, however, were found to have "*acute tubular epithelial necrosis,*"[6] a possible symptom of aspartame poisoning.

As described in "Chemical description" on page 68, about 10% of the aspartame molecule breaks down into methanol. Methanol is quickly oxidized into formaldehyde[7]—a known carcinogen, and then formic acid, a cause of kidney necrosis[8] and acute kidney failure.[9] Formic acid appears to be the principal cause of adverse effects associated with methanol poisoning.[10]

Is the FDA ADI for aspartame safe?

Note in Table 2-6 on page 2-12 that the FDA claims it is safe for a 150 lb. (68 kg) human adult (male or female) to drink up to twenty 12-oz. cans of diet soda per day. The acceptable daily intake (ADI) set for the European Union (E.U.) is 40 mg/kg,[11] or 40/50 = 0.80 = 80% of the U.S. ADI, so a 68 kg human adult in the E.U. could consume up to 16 cans of diet soda per day.

Recall from the discussion of "Dosage" on page 10 that the equivalent that a 150 lb. human male would receive in my experiment is 13 cans of diet soda per day, which is 65% of the U.S ADI and 13/16 = 0.81 or about 80% of the E.U. ADI. The equivalent that a 120 lb. (55 kg) human female would receive in my experiment is 14 cans per day, or 70% of the U.S. ADI and 14/16 = 0.875 or about 90% of the E.U. ADI.

According to the pro-aspartame authors of *The Clinical Evaluation of a Food Additive: Assessment of Aspartame*:

"The Food and Drug Act of 1906 requires that food should not contain 'any added poisonous or other added deleterious ingredient which may render such article injurious to health.' ... Accepting that no substance can be shown to be absolutely safe, the objective of safety assessment is to determine the dose of a substance at which there is reasonable certainty of no harm. To accomplish this, FDA requires extensive animal toxicity studies. From these studies, the no-observed-effect level (NOEL) or no-observed-adverse-effect level (NOAEL) is determined. To ensure reasonable certainty of no harm, FDA normally sets the ... ADI at 1% of the NOEL or NOAEL. Because NOELs or NOAELs are typically established by results from chronic toxicity or lifetime carcinogenicity studies, the ADI is the daily intake that is considered safe for an entire lifetime. If the additive is found to cause cancer in either animals or humans at any dose, it is banned from use as a food additive as a result of the Delaney Anticancer Clause of 1958."[12]

By FDA mandate, the U.S. ADI is supposed to be one-hundred times lower than the smallest amount that causes any adverse effect.

By FDA mandate, therefore, the U.S. ADI is supposed to be one-hundred times lower than the smallest amount that causes any adverse effect.

Due to the evidence documented in this report, it appears to me that both the U.S. and E.U. ADIs for aspartame are too high. In fact, it appears to me that there is no safe level of aspartame consumption. For example, if you consider the aggregate of the grossly observed adverse effects documented in this report, I believe it would be fair to state that the levels of aspartame my rats received were "*injurious to health.*"

The amount of aspartame approved for use by the FDA under its own guide-lines should therefore be at most 1/100 of the amount received by my rats.

My male rats received about 34 mg/kg/day and my females about 45 mg/kg/day. The ADI for human males should therefore be less than (34/100) mg/kg/day = 0.34 mg/kg/day. For human females, the ADI should be less than (45/100) mg/kg/day = 0.45 mg/kg/day. Recall from Table 2-1 on page 2-3, the equivalent amount of soda for human males and females would be about 13 and 14 12-oz. cans of diet soda respectively. The maximum amount of soda consumed by human males and females under these proposed aspartame ADI levels should therefore be at most 0.13 and 0.14 – 1/7 of a can of soda per day.

Is further investigation of aspartame warranted?

A friend suggested that I ask students all over the world to do their own aspartame experiments as science fair projects, and send me their data. I feel hesitant to do that. However, if you have done an experiment involving aspartame, I would be happy to post your results on my website. You can send info to me at v@writerswithoutborders.net.

Regarding the results of my experiment, I suggest that if they are ignored and the aspartame ADI remains the same, an experiment should be under-taken where diet drinks are administered at the equivalent levels given my rats to the following subjects for the rest of their lives:

The officials who got aspartame approved for public use in 1981, including Donald Rumsfeld, ex-Secretary of Defense, and then President and CEO of G.D. Searle, who used political pull to get the chemical approved in the early months of the Reagan administration;[13] Dr. Arthur Hull Hayes, who single-handedly approved aspartame at the FDA in 1981 over the objections of FDA scientists;[14] those at the FDA who over the years have refused to ban aspartame from the marketplace, though it received 77% of all complaints registered by that organization;[15] the boards of directors and officers of all aspartame manufacturers worldwide; the boards of directors and officers of all pro-aspartame organizations worldwide; and the boards of directors and officers of all manufacturers adding aspartame to more than 6,000 consum-ables worldwide.[16]

Notes

A   What is Aspartame?

"Aspartame is approximately 200 times sweeter than sugar, tastes like sugar, can enhance fruit flavors, saves calories and does not contribute to tooth decay. Products sweetened with aspartame can be useful as part of a healthful diet."

"Aspartame is approximately 200 times sweeter than sugar, tastes like sugar, can enhance fruit flavors, saves calories and does not contribute to tooth decay. Products sweetened with aspartame can be useful as part of a healthful diet."[1]

—Aspartame Information Center, industry website

"Aspartame is a molecule composed of three ingredients, aspartic acid, 40% (an excitotoxin ... that stimulates the neurons of the brain to death), ... a methyl ester that immediately converts to methyl alcohol, (10%) then breaks down to formaldehyde (embalming fluid) and formic acid (ant sting poison), and 50% phenylalanine ... a neurotoxin that lowers the seizure threshold and depletes serotonin, triggering psychiatric and behavioral problems.... The FDA lists 92 documented symptoms from aspartame, from four types of seizures and coma, to male sexual dysfunction and death."[2]

—Betty Martini, anti-aspartame activist

If you're unfamiliar with aspartame, now rebranded as AminoSweet,[3] the following pages will introduce you to this ubiquitous man-made sweetener.

Chemical classification

Aspartame is classified as an artificial, synthetic, non-nutritive, non-caloric, low-cal, low-carb, diabetic-safe and alternative-sweetener-type food additive. It is ingested by an estimated 200 million people worldwide in more than 6,000 consumables,[4] including diet sodas, fruit juices, candies, coffees, teas, pharmaceuticals, vitamins, and dairy products.

Brand names

Aspartame is marketed as a low-calorie tabletop sweetener under the names: NutraSweet,® NutraSweet Spoonfuls,® Equal,® Equal Measure,® Equal Sugar Lite,[5] Canderel,® Mivida, Sweetex, Peptis,[6] Natrasweet,®[7] NatraTaste,[8] Bienvia, Kroger Sweet Servings,[9] Sugar Twin Plus,[10] Twinsweet™,[11] Miwon,[12] Neotame,[13] Sanecta, Tri-Sweet,[14] E951,[15] NouriSweet™,[16] Aspartame,[17] and most recently, AminoSweet.[18]

Chemical description

The chemical structure of aspartame[19] is shown in Figure A-1.

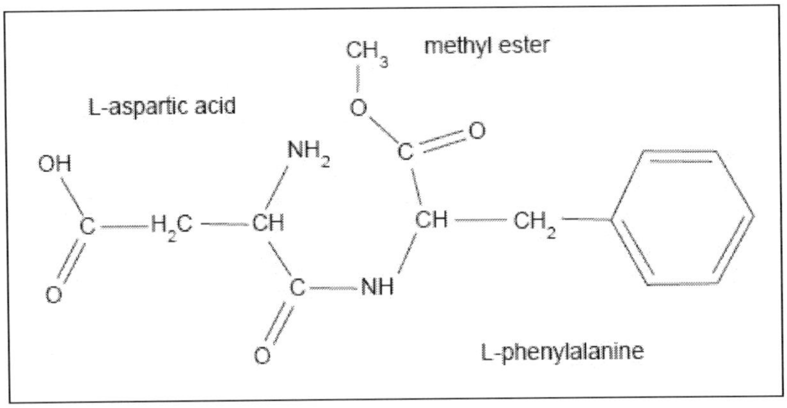

FIGURE A-1: **Chemical structure of aspartame**

Scientifically speaking, aspartame is: N-L-alpha-aspartyl-L-phenylalanine 1-methyl ester.

Aspartame's scientific name is: *N-L-alpha-aspartyl-L-phenylalanine 1-methyl ester.*[20] The name assigned to aspartame by the International Union of Pure and Applied Chemistry (IUPAC) is: *3-amino-4-(1-methoxycarbonyl-2-phenyl-ethyl) amino-4-oxo-butanoic acid.*[21] Aspartame is considered chemically synonymous with many other chemical compounds, as listed in the endnotes of this chapter.[22] Aspartame's Chemical Abstracts Service (CAS) identifier is: 22839-47-0. Its chemical formula is: $C_{14}H_{18}N_2O_5$, and its molecular mass is 294.30 g/mol.[23]

As shown in Figure A-1, the major chemical components of aspartame are:

- L-phenylalanine (CAS # 63-91-2),[24] about 50%; a biosynthetic amino acid

- L-aspartic acid (CAS # 56-84-8), about 40%; a biosynthetic amino acid

- Methyl ester, about 10%; from treating L-phenylalanine with methanol (CAS # 67-56-1, wood alcohol), in the presence of hydrochloric acid.[25]

Does Aspartame Make You Fat?

"Two-thirds of adult American women fall into the overweight or obese category."

"Two-thirds of adult American women fall into the overweight or obese category, according to their BMIs [body mass index].... *A report from the Centers for Disease Control found that the prevalence of obesity among U.S. adults doubled between 1980 and 2004 and has since stabilized at an alarmingly high level. Compared to women of a generation ago, we're 24 pounds heavier on average, and there's been an especially alarming increase in those at the upper end of the scale (not just obese, defined as a BMI of 30 or higher, but significantly obese, with a BMI above 35)."*[1]

—Barbara Kantrowitz and Pat Wingert

During my experiment, a male and female on aspartame became obese as shown in Figure 3-25 on page 37 and Figure 4-21 on page 60. None of the rats from the control group became fat. Ironically, aspartame is sold to help people lose weight. Unfortunately, it also appears to be addictive. See "Is Aspartame Addictive?" on page 75.

Aspartame and the obesity epidemic

Aspartame was introduced to the American public in dry goods starting in July of 1981, and in beverages in 1983.[2] In 2004, aspartame's meteoric rise in sales started reversing in North America. According to aspartame vendor Merisant's annual report, sales of aspartame in North America were down from $146,000,000 to $113,500,000 or 22% in 2005 over 2004, and decreased by 9.3% between 2003 and 2004.[3] The overlap in dates between the rise and stabilization of the obesity epidemic among women described in the quote at the beginning of this appendix and the rise and descent of aspartame sales in North America appear to indicate a positive correlation between the two events.

This correlation appears to be confirmed by a study from the Federal Centers of Disease Control and Prevention. A 2008 report from the Associated Press states that *"The percentage of American children who are overweight or obese appears to have leveled off after a 25-year increase, according to new figures that offer a glimmer of hope in an otherwise dismal battle.... Overall, roughly 32 percent of children were overweight but not obese, 16 percent were obese and 11 percent were extremely obese, in a study based on in-person measurements of height and weight in 2005 and 2006. The results are based on 8,165 children ages 2 to 19 who participated in nationally representative government health surveys in 2003-04 and 2005-06.... [The] levels were roughly the same as in 2003-04 after a steady rise since 1980."*[4]

By adding up the percentages of overweight and obese children in the study, we see that 59% of the children were considered overweight or obese. That appears to correlate loosely with the number of females in the CDC study, which showed that 67% of the women were overweight or obese. That stands to reason, because women probably use more diet products than children. We now need a study on men over the same time period.

Excitotoxins and weight gain

A recent study shows that each can of diet soda increases the risk of being overweight by an unbelievable 41%!

A recent study shows that each can of diet soda increases the risk of being overweight by an unbelievable 41%![5] Neurosurgeon Dr. Blaylock explains the various mechanisms that contribute to weight gain from excitotoxins such as aspartame and MSG:

"In 1969, neuroscientist Dr. John Olney discovered that feeding newborn rats MSG (monosodium glutamate) caused them to become grossly obese. Each time he repeated the experiment, he saw the same thing. Subsequent studies have shown that this phenomenon occurred in most animal species, indicating that it wasn't something peculiar to the rat. The effects of MSG are now so well established that the substance is routinely used in experimental obesity studies on animals.[6]

A study that came out in August 2008 has confirmed that the consumption of MSG causes weight gain in humans. Researchers at the University of North Carolina at Chapel Hill and in China *"studied more than 750 Chinese men and women, aged between 40 and 59, in three rural villages in north and south China. The majority of the study participants prepared their meals at home without commercially processed foods. About 82 percent of the participants used MSG in their food. Those users were divided into three groups based on the amount of MSG they used. The third who used the most MSG were nearly three times more likely to be overweight than non-users."*[7]

It's been known for more than 50 years that a tiny injury to the arcuate nucleus—part of the hypothalamus within the brain—causes gross obesity in lab animals. Scientists now know that aspartame, MSG, and other excitotoxins destroy the arcuate nucleus.[8] Dr. Blaylock has been especially concerned about infant formula. According to Blaylock:

"An intensive 1995 review of MSG toxicity by the Federation of American Societies for Experimental Biology (FASEB) concluded that infant formula contained a dose of glutamate (the toxic ingredient in MSG) in the form of caseinate (cow's milk protein) that would sufficiently produce the very same brain injury seen in experimental animals. Disturbingly humans are five times more susceptible to MSG toxicity than even the most sensitive lab animal. And babies are four times more sensitive than adults.[9]

Exposure to MSG, aspartame, and other excitotoxins in early life leads to gross obesity.[10] What's more, scientists have shown that obese animals have metabolic syndrome, defined as obesity, atherosclerosis, hypertension, and type-2 diabetes. In the U.S., about 50 million adults have metabolic syndrome.[11] According to my doctor, I am one of them.

Blaylock sums up his dismay about this situation: *"Unbelievably, dietitians, medical doctors and many public institutions are promoting the use of 'diet' soft drinks and other foods sweetened with aspartame (NutraSweet, Equal, etc.) as the answer to the problem of obesity.*[12]

How excitotoxins make us fat

Excitotoxins aspartame and MSG make us fat in several ways.

Elevation of insulin

Jack Samuels, founder of truthinlabeling.org explains on his website that: *"MSG and aspartame can cause weight gain.... When we eat foods with aspartame and/or MSG, it is now clear that it affects insulin levels, causing people to have the urge to eat more in order to balance the insulin levels. It is apparently the result of an increased level of the hormone glucagon, in the body from the excitotoxins."*[13]

> *Note: Jack Samuels maintains a website at http://www.truthinlabeling.org/hiddensources.html, that lists the hidden sources of glutamic acid, the neurotoxin in MSG. Here are the ingredients that Samuels claims always have glutamic acid: glutamate, glutamic acid, gelatin, monosodium glutamate, calcium caseinate, textured protein, monopotassium glutamate, sodium caseinate, yeast nutrient, yeast extract, yeast food, autolyzed yeast, and hydrolyzed protein. The page also lists ingredients that may contain glutamic acid or where the acid becomes present during processing, and components that may contain very small amounts of glutamic acid for those who are ultra-sensitive.*

Recent studies have shown that glutamate, the excitotoxic part of MSG and other excitotoxins such as aspartic acid from aspartame powerfully stimulate the insulin-producing cells of the pancreas.[14] According to Blaylock:

Aspartame stimulates the pancreas to secrete insulin, making you hungry, especially for sweets. The more [diet soda] *you drink, the hungrier you get."*[15]

In addition to weight gain, excess insulin causes atherosclerosis, hypertension and type-2 diabetes—the metabolic syndrome—by stimulating chronic inflammation.[16]

"Aspartame stimulates the pancreas to secrete insulin, making you hungry ... the more [diet soda] you drink, the hungrier you get."

Loss of appetite control

Leptin is a chemical produced in fat cells. It controls fat accumulation, among other things. For a normal person, when leptin enters the bloodstream, it passes the blood-brain barrier, and then enters the brain, where it acts on the arcuate nucleus to suppress the appetite and accelerate fat burning.[17] According to Blaylock:

"This vital collection of neurons [the arcuate nucleus] *is the area of the brain most sensitive to excitotoxins. In experiments, MSG rendered leptin ineffective, causing the animals to become grossly obese. Scientists call this leptin resistance, an occurrence linked to obesity in both children and adults. While*

it is soon after birth that a child may first be exposed to foods containing MSG and other excitotoxins [such as aspartame], *the effects persist for a lifetime."*[18]

Unbridled fat accumulation

Aspartame, MSG, and other excitotoxins also adversely affect fat burning, leading to fat accumulation. According to Blaylock:

"Excitotoxins like MSG [and aspartame] *cause more glucose to enter fat cells, preventing it from being burned in muscle cells as it should. As a result, more fat accumulates, especially around organs and within the abdomen. This visceral fat is the root of all the of the metabolic syndrome's bad effects.*[19]

My own morbid obesity

Recall the statistic from the beginning of this appendix: *"Two-thirds of adult American women fall into the overweight or obese category, according to their BMIs."* While consuming aspartame and MSG, I became *morbidly obese*, also referred to as *clinically severe obesity*, when one weighs more than 100 lb. (45.5 kg) over his or her ideal weight. Figure B-1 shows a slim version of myself in December 1988 at the age of 40.

Here's a photo of me in December 1988.

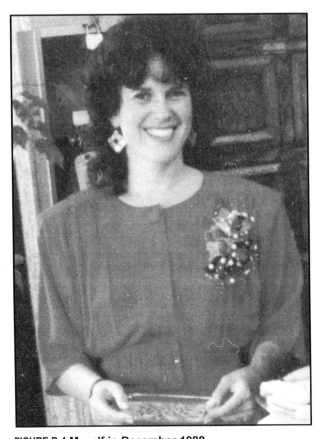

FIGURE B-1 Myself in December 1988

At that time I was *vegan*; I ate no animal products. I ate mostly raw fruits and vegetables, a diet similar to the one that brought Demi Moore at 40 into fabulous shape for the movie *Charlie's Angels—Full Throttle*.[20] I consumed no aspartame during that time.

> *Note: For one of the best books on raw foods, see* **The Raw Food Factor** *by Susan Schenck, available through the For More Info link on my website, aspartameexperiment.com.*

About a year after this photo was taken I went through a trauma from which it took several years to recover. I lost my discipline to stick to the living foods program and although I was still primarily vegetarian, I was no longer vegan. I started eating dairy products along with foods containing MSG, such as soy burgers, soy chicken patties, soy sausage links, soy bacon, and soy chorizo. I also resumed drinking diet sodas, a habit I had developed as a teenager. Figure B-2 shows a photo of me at 61, taken in December, 2009.

Here's a photo of me in December 2009.

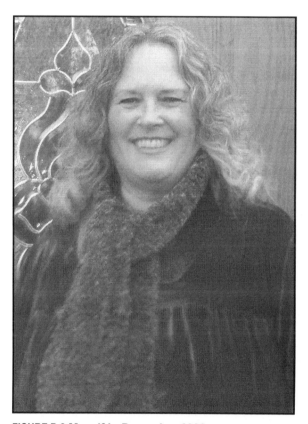

FIGURE B-2 Myself in December 2009

I have since learned that soy is almost 10% glutamic acid, the excitotoxic component of MSG. See "Soy" on page 108. I stopped drinking diet sodas in 1998, and stopped eating soy in fall of 2004. I have been struggling to lose weight with various degrees of success and failure for many years.

Notes

C

Is Aspartame Addictive?

"The wife of a man consuming up to six liters of diet cola daily concluded: 'He is truly addicted and unable to help himself.... When not drinking it, he is like a new person, or at least the person I once knew. But when he then drinks it after abstaining for a week (as a result of incredible determination), I see depression, verbal aggression, a sense of hopelessness, inability to sleep, poor concentration, trouble with eyesight, chest problems, and weight gain.'"[1]

—From an online article by H. J. Roberts, MD

What could be worse than a popular diet aid that makes you fat? One that is also addictive!

What could be worse than a popular diet aid that makes you fat? One that is also addictive! (See "Does Aspartame Make You Fat?" on page 69.)

"The anguished friend of an aspartame addict stated: 'She could hardly walk. She could hardly see. She was already going to a neurologist because they thought she had multiple sclerosis.... Her physician ... told her that aspartame was the problem, especially after he started researching its role in brain tumors—because two persons in her family died from brain tumors! When told aspartame would kill her, she said: 'I'm addicted to it and can't live without it. If they try to take it off the market, I'll get it on the black market!'"[2]

A scientist wrote the following description of alcohol addiction: "A person is said to be an alcohol addict when he or she continues to drink despite health and negative social and family problems."[3]

Substituting the word *aspartame* for *alcohol*, there is anecdotal evidence that aspartame is addictive. An article from a website for recovering alcoholics and addicts, cleanandsoberissexy.com, asks: *"Is diet soda bad for alcoholics, addicts?"*[4] The author responds:

"I had heard of several alcoholics and addicts who had been drinking large amounts of diet cola and had suffered side effects. "My friend is an alcoholic with 15 years sobriety. He said he had been drinking between 6 and 8 cans of diet cola daily for several months. He had been suffering for some time several symptoms similar to when he was drinking. All his symptoms disappeared when he stopped drinking diet cola sweetened with aspartame. His symptoms were:

- *Mood changes*
- *Depression*
- *Anxiety*
- *Anger*

- *Headaches*

- *Cloudy thinking*

- *Muscle aches and pains*

- *Tinnitus (ringing in the ears)*

- *Upset stomach*

- *Constipation*

- *Abdominal pain (left side)*

- *Poor skin tone*

- *Psoriasis (red scaly skin patches)*

- *Skin rash*

- *Frequent urination*

- *He had been told his liver and kidneys were not working effectively*

- *He often felt compelled to have the first diet cola after breakfast*

- *He often craved for the next diet cola."*

Dr. Roberts was first to draw attention to the addictive nature of aspartame. In an online article, he provides confirmation for this story when he writes: *"A previous alcoholic patient expressed concern that he had traded alcoholism for aspartame addiction. He observed in a letter: 'There are MANY just like me. You will rarely see a recovered alcoholic without a drink in hand, day or night, whether it be coffee or soda ... usually DIET. We can hardly keep sweeteners on hand at our meetings. MANY of us suffer from tremendous mood bouts. If aspartame has contributed to the difficulties I have had with depression and mood swings, I WANT TO KNOW!'"*[5]

"Recovered alcoholic patients repeatedly stated that they felt worse after avoiding aspartame than alcohol, and asserted that they had traded one addiction for another."

Dr. Roberts states that *"Thirty-three (5.6%) of 540 aspartame reactors ... found it difficult or impossible to discontinue* [diet products with aspartame] *because of severe withdrawal effects. They or their reporting relatives (especially parents of afflicted children) specifically used the terms 'addict' and 'addiction.' Others who used comparable terms were excluded even though they experienced similar withdrawal symptoms.... Recovered alcoholic patients repeatedly stated that they felt worse after avoiding aspartame than alcohol, and asserted that they had traded one addiction for another."*[6]

Two components of the aspartame molecule appear to cause the addiction: the methyl ester—about 10% of the aspartame molecule—that quickly becomes free methyl alcohol after consumption, and phenylalanine—about 50% of the molecule.

Methyl alcohol—also known as methanol, wood alcohol, carbinol, wood spirits, or wood naphtha[7]—is the most toxic form of alcohol,[8] with a smell and taste similar to ethanol.[9] It is found in windshield washer liquid and other organic solvents, gasoline, antifreeze, copy machine fluid, small stove fuel, shellac, varnish, paint strippers,[10] perfumes, and in some eau de colognes.[11] When compared to ethanol—the alcohol used in most adult beverages—methanol is only mildly intoxicating. It is, however, metabolized over a 12-to-24-hour period[12] into the highly toxic chemicals formaldehyde and formic acid, that can be responsible for headaches, cramps, convulsions, depressed breathing, acidosis, destruction of the optic nerve, permanent blindness, and death.[13] Methanol is estimated to be lethal for adults at doses of 50-100 mL (1.69-3.38 fl oz U.S.), however, blindness and death have occurred after consuming as little as 0.1 mL/kg, equivalent to about 6-10 mL, (0.20 - 0.34 fl oz U.S.) varying with the weight of the individual.[14]

A twenty-six-year old man was diagnosed with methanol poisoning. He was given ethanol to block formic acid production. He suffered two cardiac arrests and was declared brain dead. He was pronounced dead after a third cardiac arrest.

For example, a 26-year-old man was hospitalized 60 hours after ingesting a significant amount of an alcoholic beverage mixed with eau de cologne or perfume. He had complained of abdominal pain, nausea, vomiting, and blurred vision, and then lapsed into a coma. He was found to have severe metabolic acidosis, and was diagnosed with methanol poisoning, with a blood methanol of 14.6 mg/dL and formic acid content of 30 mg/L. He was given intravenous sodium bicarbonate and dialysis for the acidosis and the removal of the methanol and its metabolites. He was given ethanol to block additional formic acid production. The acidosis was eventually corrected, but he had suffered two cardiac arrests, and was declared brain dead the third day after hospitalization. He died after a third cardiac arrest.[15]

The administration of methanol to pregnant lab rats has also been shown to produce birth defects.[16]

> *Note: Folic acid, found in green leafy vegetables, is critical in the body's detoxification of methanol. When deficient, formic acid accumulates in the blood, causing acidosis. An article in the New England Journal of Medicine estimates that up to 30% of pregnant women in the United States and Europe, and 50% of pregnant women in India, have folic acid deficiencies.[17]*

According to Dr. Roberts, "*The daily intake of methyl alcohol from natural sources averages less than 10 mg. Aspartame beverages contain 55 mg methanol per liter, and nearly double as much in some carbonated orange sodas. Persons ingesting five liters* [of diet orange soda] *a day can therefore consume over 400 mg of methanol.*"[18] Food scientist and methanol expert Dr. Woodrow C. Monte calculated that a daily intake of 250 mg of methanol is 32 times the daily limit set by the Environmental Protection Agency (EPA),[19] which amounts to (250 mg/day)/32 = 7.8 mg/day. So an intake of 400 mg/day of methanol would be 400/7.8 = 51 times the EPA limit!

As you can see from the story of the man who died from methanol poisoning, ethanol is an antidote to methanol. The enzyme that metabolizes methanol—alcohol dehydrogenase—also oxidizes ethanol in the liver, and the oxidation of ethanol takes precedence over that of methanol. This allows the body to slowly excrete the methanol through the kidneys and breath with minimal formation of the deadly metabolites, formaldehyde and formic acid.[20]

Ajinomoto, the world's largest producer of aspartame, states on its website, aspartame.net, that: "*Methanol is a natural and harmless component of many foods we eat every day. The methanol produced by aspartame is identical to the methanol produced in much larger amounts from fruits, vegetables and their juices. In fact, a cup of tomato juice provides about six times more methanol than a cup of an aspartame-sweetened soft drink. The amount of methanol in the human diet is nowhere near the levels that cause toxicity. You would have to drink over 600 cans of diet soft drink at one sitting to reach the toxic level."*[21]

The problem with Ajinomoto's statement is that plant foods that naturally contain methanol also contain its antidote, ethanol. A search on the U.S. Department of Agriculture (USDA) website shows that oranges, onions, pineapple, cauliflower, tomato, and black current each contain methanol. Each of those foods also contain the antidote ethanol (also called ethyl alcohol).[22] For example, according to the USDA website, the amount of *methanol* in orange juice is between 0.8 - 80 ppm, whereas the *ethanol* content of orange juice is 64 - 900 ppm, or 11 - 80 times the methanol.[23] According to Dr. Monte in his ground-breaking work on methanol, "*Inhibition is seen in vitro even when the concentration of ethyl alcohol* [is] *only 1/16th that of methanol.*[24] *The inhibitory effect is a linear function of the log of the ethyl alcohol concentration, with a 72% inhibition rate at only a 0.01 molar concentration of ethanol. Therefore if a liter of a high methanol content orange juice is consumed, with 33 mg/liter of methanol and a 20/1 ratio of ethanol/methanol, only one molecule of methanol in 180 will be metabolized into dangerous metabolites until the majority of the ethanol has been cleared from the bloodstream.*"[25]

Aspartame contains no ethanol, and its metabolite formaldehyde, which breaks down into formic acid, has been found to collect and stay in the body after the consumption of aspartame.

Aspartame contains no ethanol, and its metabolite formaldehyde, which breaks down into formic acid, has been found to collect and stay in the body after the consumption of aspartame, as mentioned in the discussion of the Trocho study on page 59.

The case of Santiago Echiverria provides an extreme example of this phenomenon. A diabetic for fifteen to twenty years, Echiverria reportedly drank copious amounts of diet cola and coffee sweetened with Equal.

Upon his death in 1994, the funeral director found so much formaldehyde in his body that he had to close the casket because the putrid-smelling chemical was seeping through Echiverria's skin. The director was puzzled by the formaldehyde content of his body *before* arterial embalming,[26] which is done by injecting a formaldehyde solution into the jugular vein and carotid artery of the deceased.[27]

Like ethanol, methyl alcohol appears to be highly addictive. Growing evidence indicates that the dopamine D3 receptor of the nucleus accumbens (NAc)—the reward, laughter, pleasure, addiction, and fear center of the forebrain[28]—is involved in dependence on alcohol. The NAc is also where nicotine, cocaine, amphetamines, and opiates have been found to effect physical changes that make us vulnerable to addiction.[29, 30, 31] Such substances are thought to enhance dopamine neurotransmission into the NAc, but their repeated consumption leads to physical changes that reduce their initial pleasurable effects, and leave an addict wanting more.[32] Scientists have found that persistent intense dopamine transmissions into the NAc create cravings that continue long after acute symptoms of withdrawal have subsided.[33]

Withdrawal from chronic ethanol use, for example, has been found to substantially decrease dopamine neuron activity and NAc dopamine levels, resulting in long-term neuroadaptations within the dopamine systems that partially account for the high rate of relapse into alcohol-seeking behaviors, even years after drinking has stopped. Deficits in dopamine transmission in animals with a history of dependence appear to be long lasting. For example, decreased dopamine release in the NAc was found as long as two months after ethanol withdrawal.[34] Since methanol has sedative properties similar to ethanol, presumably chronic methanol consumption from sustained and frequent ingestion of aspartame results in similar dependencies.

Methanol, however, comprises approximately 10% of the breakdown derivatives of aspartame. What of phenylalanine, comprising about 50% of the molecule?

> When phenylalanine is carried to the blood-brain barrier, it competes with the amino acid tyrosine for passage into the brain. When excess phenylalanine is consumed, such as during chronic aspartame ingestion, the brain gets less and less tyrosine from food. This creates an addiction similar to that of methanol, because tyrosine is converted into the "feel-good" chemical dopamine.

Recall from our discussion of phenylalanine and aggressive behavior starting on page 48, when phenylalanine is carried to the blood-brain barrier, it competes with the amino acid tyrosine for passage into the brain. When excess phenylalanine is consumed, such as during chronic aspartame ingestion, the brain gets less and less tyrosine from food. This creates an addiction similar to that of methanol, because tyrosine is converted into the "feel-good" chemical dopamine. Continual flooding of the brain with phenylalanine results in a depletion of dopamine transmissions into the NAc, causing an addict to seek his or her drug of choice, aspartame.

Behind every craving is a powerful automated reward reinforcement system as basic as hunger or thirst. Though not fully understood, powerful internal forces affect our behaviors.[35] The healthy person achieves a balance of behaviors. We may overeat or over-indulge in alcohol or food at times, and then return to more moderate consumption. We balance the competing pleasurable reward reinforcement system and the control system that enables us to weigh the potential negative consequences.[36] Dopamine is crucial to the successful functioning of our reinforcement system. Even small amounts of chemicals that inhibit the activity of dopamine can block our reinforcement mechanisms. In one study, two groups of participants drank alcoholic beverages. One group was also given haloperidol, a drug that blocks the reception of dopamine's chemical messages of craving. The other group received a placebo. The haloperidol group consumed less alcohol.[37]

Notes

D

Misinformation About My Experiment

—Thomas Pynchon, *Gravity's Rainbow*

A website has published information about my work that is not valid, as described next in "Unauthorized website." For a description of the problems with the data on that site, see "Inaccurate information posted" on page 83.

Unauthorized website

In early 2008, a person scanned photos from an early version of this report, wrote introductory verbiage, and posted it on myaspartameexperiment.com.

In early 2008, a person scanned photos from an early version of this report, wrote introductory verbiage, and posted it on the website myaspartameexperiment.com. See Figure D-1. Note that my name appears as author at the bottom of the page.

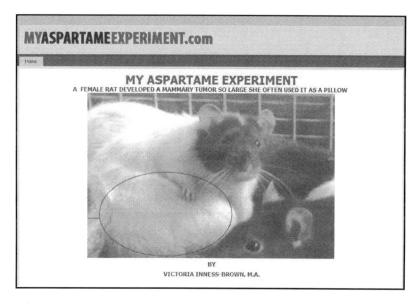

FIGURE D-1 Page 1 of myaspartameexperiment.com

Note: Content about my work was removed from this website on February 12, 2010. It still exists, however, in other locations around the web.

Figure D-2 shows a copy of a photo from page 3 of that website. If you look closely, you can see that the image was scanned from a well-worn page that appears to have been folded. Note the crease and wear marks.

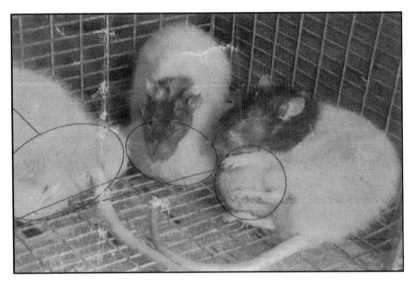

FIGURE D-2 Photo from page 3 of unauthorized website

When the website was published on February 12, 2008, I hadn't yet finished analyzing my data, and that site only presented about half of it. In addition, my protocol and data were misinterpreted. See "Inaccurate information posted" on page 83.

For the correct protocol and results of my experiment, see "My Experimental Protocol" on page 3 and "Conclusion" on page 61.

As of April 3, 2009, the unauthorized website had received over 220,000 hits, according to an e-mail from its author. The website led to passionate discussions about my work on the popular blogs reddit.com and digg.com, and numerous smaller blogs and websites. See "What They Say About My Experiment" on page 85.

A few days after the website was brought online, a stranger sent me a message about the blog activity. I read through the blogs with intensely mixed feelings. After considering the situation and getting advice from others supporting my work, I decided not to respond to anything, and to lay low until my report was ready for publication.

I finished analyzing my data in summer of 2008 and opened my official website aspartameexperiment.com in September 2008. See Figure D-3. There you can see an overview of this report and its photos.

I published the first color edition of this report electronically through my website at that time.

> I finished analyzing my data in summer of 2008 and opened my official website aspartameexperiment.com in September 2008.

Misinformation About My Experiment   My Aspartame Experiment—

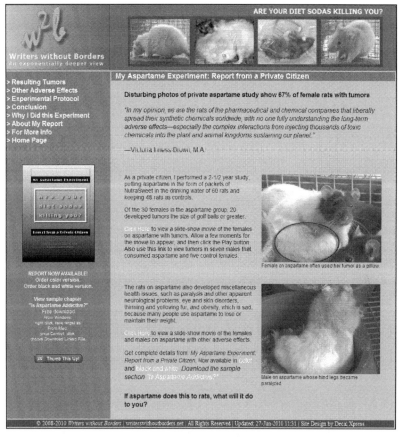

FIGURE D-3 **My official website, aspartameexperiment.com**

As I prepared to send the print version to the publishing house, however, I was advised to make further modifications. I eliminated access to the electronic version and continued to work on the report. The changes have taken over a year, resulting in a significantly larger work, with most of the new information presented in Appendices B through F.

Inaccurate information posted

The unauthorized website, myaspartameexperiment.com, was based on incomplete data.

As mentioned earlier, the unauthorized website, myaspartameexperiment.com, was based on incomplete data. The inaccuracies are explained in the following subsections.

Incorrect tumor rates

Page 2 of that site incorrectly reports these tumor rates: *"Eleven females and one male developed tumors. That's 37% of the females on aspartame."*

As described in "Tumors in my aspartame group" on page 62, upon completion of my data analysis, I found that 20 out of 30, or 67% of my females on aspartame developed tumors, and 7 out of 30, or 23% of my males on aspartame developed tumors.

Victoria Inness-Brown, M.A.   83

In addition, page 7 of the unauthorized website inaccurately states the following in a footnote:

"Three female rats in the control group of 48 had small tumors."

Actually 5 out of 24, or 21% of my control females developed tumors that were generally smaller than those in the females on aspartame. None of my control males developed tumors.

Incorrect equivalencies of diet soda

The unauthorized website states that the amount of aspartame I gave my rats was equivalent to a single can of diet soda per day if my experiment were repeated on humans. The actual value is less impressive. My calculations for the equivalent cans of soda are provided in "Dosage" on page 10.

The results of the calculations show that for a 150 lb. (68 kg) human male, the equivalent would be about 13 cans, or 2.25 two-liter bottles of diet soda per day.

For a 120 lb. (54.5 kg) human female, the equivalent would be about 14 cans, or 2.4 two-liter bottles of diet soda per day.

Page two of the unauthorized website inaccurately states that:

"To put these numbers into perspective, the aspartame received by my rats daily, was equivalent to two-thirds the aspartame contained in 8-oz of diet soda."

The correct statement is more complex. Please see "Dosage" on page 10 for cross references. Since each 8 oz. of drinking water in my experiment contained about 80 mg of aspartame, the aspartame was equivalent to about 80 mg / 120 mg = 0.67 = 67%—or two-thirds the aspartame contained in 8 oz. of diet soda. The aspartame received by my rats was therefore equivalent to their receiving about two-thirds of their daily fluid as diet soda and the remainder as water.

E

What They Say About My Experiment

"It's obvious she did her best to make this experiment as close to a real scientific study as possible and its effects are very eye opening. I would like to see this experiment repeated by real (unbiased) professionals now two or three more times. If the results are similar then we may have a serious problem with this sweetener. I admit I drink diet soda as well but I may cut back or stop now. Coffee has been a big help in weaning myself from sugar/artificial sweeteners while still getting my caffeine fix."[1]

—Poster unknown

Quotes from the controversy

The unauthorized website myaspartameexperiment.com is not my website and some of its data is incorrect. See "Misinformation About My Experiment" on page 81.

> The author generated lots of publicity for the site, evoking intense controversy, resulting in my name appearing in a number of blogs and more than 2000 websites.

Though it's not my website, it shows many of my photos and discusses my experiment *as if I were the author*. The actual author generated lots of publicity for the site, evoking intense controversy, resulting in my name appearing in a number of mainstream blogs and more than 2000 websites.

Here is a sprinkling of the responses:

"Greetings from Pori, west coast of Finland. I saw your aspartame experiment first in Mercola's blog and I want to thank you for your incredible work, those pictures truly say more than a thousand words."[2]

—Marjo Sukeva

"I came across your "My Aspartame Experiment" and I had to write you to let you know that my wife and I appreciate what you have done. At the same time I'm sorry that you even had to do the experiment. We all should have known better. It didn't have to be put in our food and drinks. But here we are in this world and people like you are doing what you can to make it a better place. We are thankful for you. May God bless you and keep you ... We were wondering how things went with your family. Did they stop drinking diet drinks in the end? It would be wonderful to hear how things went for you and your family."[3]

—Edward

Note: For news about the effect my experiment had on my family's consumption of diet soda with aspartame, see "Update to article in Smart Money magazine" on page 89.

see "Update to article in Smart Money magazine" on page 89.

"*This website is astounding. Victoria Inness-Brown, M.A. did research for all of us and for all our children.*"

"This website is astounding. Victoria Inness-Brown, M.A. did research for all of us and for all our children."[4]

—Scaredhuman

"I am French Canadian and with a friend who lives in France and who will accept to give me a help hand, we will translate into French your aspartame experiment. The French translation will be for sure published on www.alter-info.net, a popular French Web site which published several articles usually not published by the mainstream media.

"I want to get your authorisation ... because the article http://www.myaspartameexperiment.com/index.php?page=1 is copyrighted and, if you agree, the French version will be posted without copyright as it is always the case for articles published on Alter Info.

Thank you and thank you for having done that experiment.

God bless you.

—Dany Quirion, Quebec city

Giving up Aspartame. On this date, Feb. 15, 2008, I have poured out 20 oz. of Diet Coke into the drain. I weigh 213 pounds at 6'1". After reading about a private aspartame experiment, and recalling similar readings, I have decided that I am switching to a water-based diet, and for the next year will not eat foods containing artificial sweeteners. I will not change my eating habits in any other way. Rather than buy 'sugar-free' jello or pudding (and similar products), I will continue to eat those products with the normal sugar content. I will also not change my exercise regimen of 'occasional' work-outs. Completely non-experimentally sound (as it also means giving up the caffeine and carbonation in the diet sodas), I want to see what happens to my weight and health over the next year. I will post on my progress if anything interesting occurs (like losing that 20-30 pounds I'm carrying around needlessly).[5]

—Rich

"You're in my Mercola newsletter this morning! I saw the headline 'One Woman's Astonishing Experiment with Aspartame' and thought 'Great, I'll forward it to Victoria,' and then discovered it's about you!"[6]

—Lalchumi Ralte

"Your hideous, cruel AT-HOME experiment on rats are inapplicable to humans and the deliverance of inexcusable cruelty. While I do not for a minute doubt that aspartame, as they say, is dangerous to humans, the proper studies would be clinical and epidemiological studies on humans. You are the same as Frankenstein!"[7]

—Diane M. Kaste

"Uh, animal studies are what the FDA is supposed to rely upon before they allow a new food or drug to be approved. The Delaney clause requires any additive that is found to cause cancer in lab animals, to be banned. The FDA broke the law when they allowed aspartame on the market. They had the data back then showing it caused brain tumors in rats and they ignored it. Aspartame is a dangerous drug."[8]

—canUdi9it

"While I'm no advocate of aspartame, this experiment is highly illegal. A person can't just start their own experiment involving animals. What if someone wants to know how many cigarettes a dog can smoke before it dies?"[9]

—cubicledropout

*"I like how if a person does it on a small scale it's highly illegal. If a corporation does it on a massive scale it's for the 'greater good' or some *****. I have to wonder what qualifications/conditions one must meet to get the permit to kill animals for science. And in this case, is it really animal cruelty if the substance used is 'okay' for a healthy human diet? Cigarettes are an obvious bad thing, because cigarettes are proven unhealthy."[10]*

—scooterbaga

"I think what most people want is the ability for private scientists to perform experiments."

"The problem is that corporations can sway the results of any study and all the news will report is 'A major study' and not the details. I think what most people want is the ability for private scientists to perform experiments. That doesn't mean that it shouldn't be regulated but still an available option. Also this particular experiment is garbage, 80 mg of aspartame is an insane quantity for a rat. That's like a human eating a pound a day. I'm willing to bet that a pound of sugar would do the same to a human."[11]

—r00k1200

> **Note: These statistics were misrepresented on *myaspartameexperiment.com*, which claims that the rats received an equivalent of less than a can of diet soda per day. See "Inaccurate information posted" on page 83.**

"That's right it's illegal to find out the truth on your own. Trust and depend on the findings of others that are free of outside influences. ;-|"[12]

—dimplemonkey

"I don't see the difference in using rats in an experiment or breaking their neck to be fed to a snake. In both cases they die. Honestly, developing a tumor is probably less painful than grabbing a rat by the tail and smacking it on the ground to break their neck. I've worked at a pet store with some large snakes that refused to eat anything live, so this is what had to be done."[13]

—lik3n

"Illegal to feed rats something that is legal for human consumption? Is there even an ounce of logic in that?"[14]

—JohnBoyer

"'I strongly believed the artificial sweetener might one day lead to their illness and even early death. I was convinced I would see tumors and possibly other harmful effects to convince my family and friends to avoid aspartame. Gee, can you say 'confirmation bias'?"[15]

—kyle90

"Yes but the data is well reported. If her experiment was carried as shown then I see a possibility of correlation. Further study is needed for causation."[16]

—chemicalwahoo

"Ha-ha. Data is well reported? Grainy pictures of god knows what? Half dead looking rats? No autopsy's? No actual tests done? Its half assed, not scientific at all, with no way of knowing what is true or not. When I was in grade 5 I did better scientific studies than this idiot."[17]

—snugglebear

> **Note: As mentioned in this report, my purpose was to document any visually obvious adverse effects. I never claimed to do a rigorous study.**

"Wanting rats to have tumors from consuming aspartame doesn't make it happen."

—Fratz

"Yes, but a vested interest in interpreting the experimental data to get a certain conclusion means a lack of scientific discipline."

—nonsequitor

"Data is data. Lots of scientists have expectations about the outcomes of experiments, especially when testing physics theories. The expectation doesn't change the data."

—Fratz

Update to article in Smart Money magazine

An excellent article about my work by award-winning journalist Anne Kadet appeared in *Smart Money* magazine in September, 2008.

An excellent article about my work by award-winning journalist Anne Kadet appeared in *Smart Money* magazine in September, 2008. See http://www.smartmoney.com/personal-finance/health-care/aspartame-safe/. I'd like to make a small update to the information in that article.

The end of the article says *"Of course, her family is still drinking diet soda. While amateurs are gaining ground on the experts these days, it's still true that no one listens to their mother."*

My step father died a terrible death after being diagnosed with a stomach tumor. Though I showed him the photos in this report, he continued to consume aspartame until a few days before his death.

I'm pleased to say, however, that the family member who most inspired my experiment (who has a scientific background and wishes to remain anonymous) told me after reading a prerelease version of this book: *"By the way, your report is very convincing. I've cut way down on drinking diet sodas with aspartame."*

Notes

F

Did I Fake My Data?

"The greatest scientists in history are great precisely because they broke with consensus. There is no such thing as consensus science. If it's consensus, it isn't science. If it's science, it isn't consensus."

"Let's be clear: the work of science has nothing whatever to do with consensus. Consensus is the business of politics. Science, on the contrary, requires only one investigator who happens to be right, which means that he or she has results that are verifiable by reference to the real world. In science consensus is irrelevant. What is relevant is reproducible results. The greatest scientists in history are great precisely because they broke with consensus. There is no such thing as consensus science. If it's consensus, it isn't science. If it's science, it isn't consensus. Period."[1]

—Michael Crichton

I published a color edition of this report electronically via my website aspartameexperiment.com in September 2008. As I prepared to send the print version to be published, however, I was advised to make further modifications. As a result, I took the electronic version down and continued to work on the report. This appendix was written as part of that process.

Why I wrote this appendix

"Unauthorized website" on page 81 describes a site about my work that caused a stir on the Internet in February 2008. After that website came out, one person blogged that I had obviously faked my data because my control group had so few health problems. On reading that, I thought about why my control group might have been healthier than most. I formed various hypotheses to answer that question and researched them one by one. You'll find my analyses in "Why was my control group relatively healthy?" on page 114.

I was, in fact, upset when I started observing tumors in my control group females, and thought my experiment a failure. My control group consisted of the older rats that I had raised. I had become fond of them, and didn't want to give them aspartame. I believe their age caused them to start getting tumors earlier in the experiment than the females on aspartame, most of whom developed tumors as they matured. I was naive in thinking my control group shouldn't have any tumors. Control groups in many published aspartame studies have had them. In any case, for my analyses of possible causes, see "What may have caused my control group tumors?" on page 99.

Though the unauthorized website described only about half my data, the results were still astounding to many people. See "What They Say About My Experiment" on page 85. After I finished analyzing my data I calculated an astronomical tumor rate of 67% for my females on aspartame—almost twice the 37% tumor rate stated on the unauthorized website. See "Inaccurate information posted" on page 83. I imagined people might find my actual tumor rate unbelievable, so I presented photos of the 20 out of 30 females on aspartame that had visible tumors on my website, aspartameexperiment.com. I wondered why I obtained such extreme results. I again came up with hypothetical answers and researched them one by one. See what I found in "Why so many tumors in my females on aspartame?" on page 93. I know of no other experiment with such a huge number of tumors in its females on aspartame. I believe that it was primarily because no other experiment put aspartame in the rats' drinking water, forcing them to ingest it. As a result, I believe that more of the breakdown components of aspartame got into their blood streams. See "Consumption of aspartame in liquid form" on page 94.

In addition, I believe that some of the same reasons that my control females developed tumors also applied to my females on aspartame, especially when you consider the multiplicative effect of numerous toxins in the body. See "Chemical cocktails multiply toxic effects" on page 99.

I was advised not to publish the information in this appendix, as it may appear that other factors caused the tumors for my females on aspartame. I want to emphasize, however, that *the only difference in treatment between my control and experimental groups was the administration of aspartame.* So in my opinion, it was the aspartame that brought about the significant number of tumors and other adverse effects in my experimental group.

I wrote the section "Females on aspartame had three times more tumors than males" shown next, before I researched the information presented in the other sections of this appendix. In it, I state that I believe aspartame may be estrogenic. After completing the research described in this appendix, I feel even stronger that this hypothesis may be true. Perhaps someone in the pharmaceutical industry might test it and report back to us. In fact, drugs mimicking estrogen, called xenoestrogens, are a common theme throughout this appendix. The primary effect of estrogen in females appears to be mammary tumors, which are prevalent throughout my data. See "Tumors in my aspartame group" on page 24.

> I found much of the cited research truly frightening, especially the section on "GM food" on page 102.

As you read this appendix, it may scare you. I found much of the cited research truly frightening, especially the section on "GM food" on page 102. Doing this research has woken me up and may have extended my life. It inspired me to become more stringent in eating a whole-food, plant-based, organic-food diet; drinking pure water, organic white tea, and various herbal teas; adding new supplements to my diet, avoiding toxic substances as much as possible, and doing something about the high estrogen levels in my body.

Females on aspartame had three times more tumors than males

The total number of rats with tumors in my aspartame group was 27, consisting of 20 females and 7 males. The percentage of females in the aspartame group with tumors was therefore 20/27 = 74%; while the percentage of males was 7/27 = 26%. My females on aspartame therefore experienced 20/7 = 2.857 or 286% more tumors than their male counterparts. This coincides with Dr. Roberts' observation that females are more affected by aspartame than males by a 3:1 ratio, as the ratio of tumors in females-to-males in my experiment was also essentially 3:1.

In his 1000+ page opus, *Aspartame Disease: An Ignored Epidemic*, H.J. Roberts, MD, describes how males and females are affected differently by aspartame in his case studies:

> *"Women* [on aspartame] *consistently outnumbered men within every subgroup* [of adverse effects] *by a 3:1 ratio. In its monitoring of adverse reactions to aspartame products, the FDA also reported that 77% of complainants were female* [a 3:1 ratio]. *In this group, 76% were between 20 and 59 years [of age], and 10% less than 20 years* [of age]."[2]

"Women [on aspartame] consistently outnumbered men within every sub-group [of adverse effects] by a 3:1 ratio."

My calculations also coincide with the number of complaints about aspartame from females reporting to the FDA (before it stopped accepting them), who registered 77% of all complaints. That's close to the value I calculated of 74% my females with observed tumors compared to 26% of my males.

Do women consume more diet products than men? Possibly. I read some-where that no matter how out of shape men are, many think that they look great. (Good for them!) Whereas, no matter how fit women are, they often feel that their appearance is lacking.

Self-image notwithstanding and for reasons unknown, the females in my study consumed more aspartame per body weight than the males. They con-sumed on average about 45 mg/kg per day, while the males consumed about 33.8 mg/kg. The males therefore ingested about 33.8/45 = 75% of the aspar-tame per body weight as the females.

Though the difference in consumption may partially explain why my females developed more tumors than my males on aspartame, it doesn't explain why my females developed three times the tumors. Let's do the math. If n is the number of females with tumors, and 7 males develop tumors while consuming 75% of the aspartame consumed by the females, we have $7 = 0.75\,n$, or $n = 7/(0.75) = 9$. If consumption were to be the only factor, then only 9 of my females on aspartame would have developed tumors. However 20 females developed tumors, more than twice the predicted number! Based on this calculation, it appears that females are at least 200% more affected by aspartame than males.

This leads me to believe that aspartame affects female hormones, and is probably estrogenic. According to *The Rat: An Owner's Guide to a Happy Healthy Pet*, neutering can *"keep them from getting uterine, mammary, or ovarian cancer."*[3] So neutering appears to prevent cancer of the female organs. Throughout this appendix, you'll find the hormone estrogen and can-cer of the female organs to be a recurring theme.

Why so many tumors in my females on aspartame?

A 67% tumor rate among females on aspartame is almost three times the rate observed in the Soffritti studies. Why did my females on aspartame have such a high tumor rate? In my opinion, it's mostly due to the design of my study, as discussed in "Consumption of aspartame in liquid form" and "My study was continued until the death of my rats" on page 94. Subsequent subsections explore other possible reasons.

Consumption of aspartame in liquid form

The aspartame consumption of choice for my family was diet soda. In fact, two-thirds of the yearly consumption of aspartame in the U.S. is from diet drinks. I thought it important to simulate diet soda consumption, and dissolved aspartame in the form of NutraSweet in with my rats' drinking water, thereby forcing them to consume it. I provided a mixture I thought would be equivalent to the aspartame in diet soda. I hadn't done the calculations at that time, however, and was off by a factor of two. Most diet sodas contain more than twice the aspartame than that contained in the water my rats received. See "Dosage" on page 10.

Aspartame in solution is absorbed much faster and more completely by the body as opposed to aspartame in solids or capsules.

What does this have to do with the high tumor rate? Aspartame in solution is absorbed much faster and more completely by the body as opposed to aspartame in solids or capsules. See the discussion in "Liquid or solid?" on page 6. Most animal studies mix aspartame crystals in dry food, and double-blind human studies provide aspartame in capsules.

The use of dry food is necessary in animal studies because of the high amounts of aspartame used, because it is difficult to maintain large amounts in solution. It becomes a thick slurry that tends to precipitate out and must constantly be shaken or stirred. Placing aspartame crystals in dry food presents other problems as well, as discussed in *The Bressler Report*, the inspiration for my experiment. For example, aspartame crystals can clump or fall to the bottom of the mixture, and thereby be avoided. In the case of the food I gave my rats, this would certainly have been the case, as it consisted of whole grains and other large food particles such as alfalfa pellets.

Double-blind studies in humans administer aspartame in capsules to prevent participants from noticing its sweet taste. Capsules take longer to dissolve and their contents are metabolized more slowly than aspartame taken alone. In fact, if a subject's digestion is poor, the capsules may be excreted from the body whole. In that case, none of the content is absorbed.

To my knowledge, only one other study added aspartame to the drinks of its subjects. That was a primate study undertaken by Harry Waisman, MD. In Waisman's experiment, aspartame was added to milk ingested by seven monkeys. One of them died after 300 days, and five of them developed seizures.[4] In addition to milk, the monkeys had pure water to drink. They were not forced to consume aspartame and may have avoided it.

My study was continued until the death of my rats

The Waisman study was stopped after 15 months. Yet the average lifespan of a monkey is 13 years = 156 months. (The maximum lifespan is 29 years.)[5] The effects of the additive were therefore observed in that study for less than 10% of the primates' average lifetime. My study, like the Soffritti studies, was done until the natural deaths of my subjects. And like Soffritti, I found that most tumors appeared in the last third of their lifetimes.

Most of the other studies I've seen were very short term and those studies labeled "long-term" ended at around two years, so they eliminated the possibility of discovering tumors and other adverse affects that might have appeared during the subjects' old age.

The longest studies cited were less than 1% of an average person's 70-year lifetime. Many lasted a week! Some only 24 hours!

In 1996 Monsanto was the primary manufacturer of aspartame. (According to monsanto.com, "*In 2000, the NutraSweet Company was sold to J.W. Childs and Equal was sold to Merisant.*") In 1996, however, a group of Monsanto scientists compiled a book to prove the safety of the additive. *The Clinical Evaluation of a Food Additive: Assessment of Aspartame* cited numerous groups of human studies. Yet the longest studies cited were less than 1% of an average person's 70-year lifetime. Many lasted only a week! Some only 24 hours! See Table 2-8, "Duration of human studies proving the safety of aspartame in 1996," on page 15. In quotes throughout this report, however, you'll find that people often started having adverse effects only after many years of consumption. In my opinion, none of the cited studies evaluated the long-term chronic use of the synthetic sweetener in humans.

I've seen the lack of pharmaceutical studies in the elderly human population as well. In December 2008, my step-father died a very unpleasant death at the age of 91. During his final months, I used rxlist.com to research the adverse effects of the prescription drugs he was on, as he appeared to suffer horrendously from them. For example, his cardiologist kept him on a high dose of blood thinner that caused internal bleeding and nearly killed him in January, 2008. That doctor also prescribed digitalis that was recalled by its manufacturer a few months later due to mislabeling. During the time he took it, he was getting twice the prescribed dosage of that dangerous drug. Without describing its adverse effects or providing any other options, my Dad's oncologist prescribed chemotherapy for him in February 2008 for a slow-growing tumor that might have killed him in five years. It is ironic to me that his stated cause of death was cancer.

During those difficult months, I read about the drugs he was taking, including the summaries of the safety studies done for each drug. Not once did I find that a drug had been tested on people my Dad's age. Yet drugs routinely given to the elderly affect them more intensely than younger folks. Geriatric patients often have limited food and liquid intake, limited kidney function, low body weight, and do minimal physical exercise, so the drugs given them affect them more than younger people. Just as Soffritti studies rats until their deaths, so human studies should be continued into our older years so that we may understand how drugs affect us throughout old age.

Possible non-inert components of NutraSweet

As mentioned in "Diet Pepsi, aspartame or NutraSweet?" on page 5, I found it difficult to purchase pure aspartame for my study, and instead used packets of NutraSweet, the tabletop sweetener made from aspartame.

The NutraSweet label states that its ingredients are aspartame, dextrose and maltodextrin. I thought the non-aspartame ingredients would be inert, with no effect on the health of my rats. Now I'm not sure. According to Jack Samuels, author of truthinlabeling.org, maltodextrin may contain MSG, possibly because of the way it is processed.[6]

"Excitotoxins have been found to dramatically promote cancer growth and metastasis. When you increase the glutamate level, cancer just grows like wildfire, and then when you block glutamate, it dramatically slows the growth of the cancer."

The glutamate (or glutamic acid) component of MSG may impair our immune systems, making us more susceptible to cancer and other diseases. In 1992, the journal *International Immunology* reported elevated blood glutamate levels in individuals testing positive for the AIDS virus (HIV-1) and suffering from depletion of T4+ T cells. High glutamate levels have also been found in cancer patients.[7] In a September 2009 online article, neurosurgeon Dr. Russell Blaylock is quoted as saying *"Excitotoxins have been found to dramatically promote cancer growth and metastasis. When you increase the glutamate level, cancer just grows like wildfire, and then when you block glutamate, it dramatically slows the growth of the cancer."*[8]

Elevated glutamate levels inhibit the membrane transport of cystine, causing an intracellular decrease of the amino acid.[9] Cystine supports healthy immune function by building up white blood-cells.[10] HIV-1 infected persons with low glutamate and high cystine levels have the highest T cell counts and lymphocyte reactivity. Patients with lung cancer, low glutamate, and high cystine levels have a longer mean survival time.[11]

Note: Green tea may help protect you against MSG. It contains from 5,000 to 13,500 ppm[12] of the amino acid theanine, which is structurally similar to glutamate, and acts as a competitive antagonist at glutamate receptors, preventing the associated neurons from firing.[13,14]

Perhaps theanine is part of the reason that animal and in vitro studies have shown that green tea may reduce the risk of UV-induced skin cancer, as well as gastro-intestinal, colon, lung, breast and ovarian cancer. Green tea may also inhibit the proliferation of leukemia, cervical and prostate cancer. It has also been found to inhibit the proliferation of head, neck, and pancreatic carcinoma cells. Additional possible benefits of theanine include improved mood and learning ability, and reduced anxiety, blood pressure, cholesterol, and weight.[15]

White, green, and black teas are made from the same plant, the camelia sinensis, by harvesting it at different stages of growth and processing it using different methods.[16] According to the USDA Phytochemical and Ethnobotanical Database website white, green, and black teas have the following phytochemicals that help prevent cancer: alanine, catechin, cinnamic-acid, epicatechin, epicatechin-gallate, glycine, hypoxanthine, isovitexin, methyl-salicylate, myricetin, niacin, o-cresol, p-cresol, pantothenic-acid, phenol, quercetin-3-o-beta-glucoside, riboflavin, safrole, serine, and vitexin.

The database states that the following phytochemicals in camelia sinensis can help reverse cancer: alpha-terpineol, benzaldehyde (tumors), butyric-acid (tumors), epigallocatechin-gallate (tumors), farnesol (pancreatic cancer), lutein (breast cancer, breast and colon tumors), malic-acid (tumors), and zeaxanthin (breast cancer, tumors).

The database also states that camelia sinensis has the following phytochemicals that help both prevent and reverse cancer: apigenin (lung cancer, and lung, breast, and skin tumors), ascorbic-acid (gastric and lung

Note (cont.): tumors), beta-carotene (breast, central nervous system, colon, lung, prostate, and stomach tumors), beta-ionone (tumors), caffeic-acid (skin tumors), caffeine (lung tumors), chlorogenic-acid (colon, fore-stomach, liver, and skin cancer), cysteine (tumors), gallic-acid (tumors), geraniol (pancreatic tumors), hyperoside, isoquercitrin (tumors), kaempferol (tumors), lycopene (bladder, breast, cervix, prostate, cancer and tumors), naringenin (tumors), polyphenols (tumors), quercetin (bladder, breast, colon, lung, ovary, and skin tumors), quercitrin (tumors), rutin, and salicylic-acid (tumors).[17]

Regarding weight loss, a report cited in the American Journal of Clinical Nutrition stated that "green tea extract resulted in a significant increase in energy expenditure." Energy expenditure is a measure of metabolism. Increasing your metabolism is one way to lose weight.[18]

There is risk involved in drinking tea, however.

There is risk involved in drinking tea, however. Some brands are high in fluoride and aluminum. Those made from older tea leaves are not only higher in these toxins, but have smaller amounts of beneficial nutrients.

Caution: You may want to restrict your tea consumption to brands of organic white tea only, with no lemon. Tea leaves have been found to accumulate fluoride from the water, soil, pesticides,[19] and herbicides in their environment more than any other plant.[20,21] (For more about the risks of fluoride, see "Fluoride in tap water" on page 117.) A study from Zhejiang University, People's Republic of China found the fluoride content in commercial teas to increase with the age of the crop.

White tea is harvested from buds and young leaves and contains the least amount of fluoride. Green tea is made from fully developed leaves and has more fluoride. Black tea is made from the more mature leaves[22] and contains from 10 to 20 times the fluoride of young leaves from the same plant.[23] In a Polish study, adults and children drinking five cups of black tea a day were found to consume up to 303% of that country's measure of the Safe and Adequate Daily Intake (SAI) of fluoride.[24] Brick tea, made from the oldest leaves and shaped into a brick, has the highest fluoride content. Tibetans drinking large amounts of brick tea have developed dental fluorosis, a permanent mottling and browning of the teeth, symptomatic of the overconsumption of fluoride.[25]

Fluoride often occurs naturally in soil and rock, and the run-off goes into the groundwater. Fluoride pollution is also caused by run-off from ashes of fluoride-rich coal burned or disposed of on open ground. Such pollution has become a major problem in China, affecting the drinking water of over 62,000,000 people.[26] In India, the groundwater of approximately 65% of the villages is polluted with fluoride.[27] This is bad news for tea drinkers worldwide, because China and India are global leaders in tea production. Their combined harvest in 2007 was 2,132,722 tons, or 55% of the worldwide market.[28]

Caution (cont.): Iced tea mixes and some decaffeinated brands have even higher amounts of fluoride, possibly due to processing with fluoridated water. In 2005, WebMD reported that commercial iced tea mixes were found with up to 6.5 parts per million (ppm) of fluoride. Yet the maximum allowed by the U.S. Environmental Protection Agency (EPA) in drinking water is 4 ppm, while the FDA restricts fluoride in beverages to 2.4 ppm.[29] When brewed in tap water at restaurants, homes, and businesses in fluoridated communities, even greater amounts of fluoride are consumed. Extended brewing times also increase the fluoride content of tea beverages.[30]

In addition to finding a positive correlation between the age of tea leaves at harvest and fluoride content, the Zhejiang study found a negative correlation between the age of tea leaves at harvest and the content of beneficial phytochemicals—the older the tea leaves at harvest, the fewer phytochemicals in the resulting tea.[31] This may result from the processing of each type of tea. White tea is the least processed, green tea is more processed, and black tea is the most highly processed.

In contrast, an independent study sponsored by Traditional Medicinals found the company's organic green tea to be fluoride free.[32] Though some may question the independence of this study, it stands to reason that teas grown without fluoride-laced chemical pesticides, herbicides, and fertilizers would have smaller amounts of fluoride.

In addition to accumulating fluoride as they age, tea leaves accumulate aluminum from their environment.[33] Neurosurgeon Dr. Blaylock reports that aluminum has been associated with Alzheimer's, and possibly Parkinson's and Lou Gehrig's diseases.[34] Blaylock therefore warns against adding lemon to your tea. According to him, "Studies have shown that little of the aluminum in tea is absorbed by the body because it is bound by catechins (flavonoids) in the tea. Yet, squeezing lemon in tea dramatically increases aluminum absorption, somewhere close to 700 percent. Flavor your tea with mint instead." Blaylock also recommends that you only drink white tea.[35]

According to Samuels, the NutraSweet ingredient dextrose may also have small or trace amounts of MSG sufficient to effect those with extreme MSG sensitivity.[36] The website drugs.com lists the following adverse effects for dextrose: "*Severe allergic reactions (rash; hives; difficulty breathing; tightness in the chest; swelling of the mouth, face, lips, or tongue); confusion; muscle twitching; seizures; swelling of the hands or feet; weakness.*"[37]

Both the maltodextrin and dextrose from NutraSweet may therefore have weakened the immune systems of my rats, making them more vulnerable to developing tumors and other adverse effects. In addition, both maltodextrin and dextrose are usually made from corn that may have been genetically modified,[38] introducing a wild card into the equation. See "GM food" on page 102.

Continual exposure to ambient noise

My rats were housed outside, near a noisy air compressor that ran an Amish air pump used to irrigate fruit trees and gardens. The pump ran much of the time most days during my experiment.

According to Bart Kosko, author of *Noise*, *"Noise can cause stress, ... [it] can disrupt or even prevent sleep—and sleep loss promotes stress and a variety of health problems from increased blood pressure to decreased immune response...."*[39]

So the noise from the compressor may have affected the immune systems of my rats, making them more susceptible to disease.

Chemical cocktails multiply toxic effects

As described throughout this appendix, my rats may were exposed to multiple toxins and environmental stressors, possibly resulting in higher tumor rates. The Soil Association reported on a three-year study of the effects of combining food additives that seems to confirm this hypothesis. The report describes research from the University of Liverpool that examined the toxic effects on nerve cells from a combination of these four food additives:

- E133 (brilliant blue)

- E621 [monosodium glutamate (MSG)]

- E104 (quinoline yellow)

- E951 [L-aspartyl-L-phenylalanine methyl ester (aspartame)]

> The adverse effects were up to ... seven times greater when quinoline yellow and aspartame were combined. The combination was found to stop nerve cells from normal growth and interfere with central nervous system (CNS) signalling systems.

They found that mixtures of the additives had a multiplicative effect, resulting in far more potent adverse effects on nerve cells when compared with the sums of the results of each additive on its own. For example, the adverse effects were up to four times greater when brilliant blue and MSG were combined, and up to seven times greater when quinoline yellow and aspartame were combined. Both combinations were found to stop nerve cells from normal growth and interfere with central nervous system (CNS) signalling systems. The additives were combined to reflect the compounds entering the bloodstream from the consumption of children's snacks and drinks. The Soil Association identified a total of 30 foods marketed to children that include the four additives.[40]

My rats were exposed to multiple chemicals, including those from NutraSweet, as well as pesticides and herbicides. The chemical cocktail they received probably resulted in far more tumors than if aspartame were the only chemical they ingested.

What may have caused my control group tumors?

As discussed in "Tumors in my control group" on page 62, five females and no males in my control group developed tumors. The percentage of tumors in the female control group was 21%, compared to 67% of my females on aspartame.

Far fewer of the rats in my control group developed any of the other adverse effects observed in my aspartame group. See "Other adverse effects in my aspartame group" on page 62 and "Other adverse effects in my control group" on page 62.

I believe there are reasons why people develop tumors. Norm Sakow, DC, raised hundreds of rats. He is a raw food vegan (a vegetarian who eats no animal products). He fed his rats the same food he ate, and claims that *none of his rats developed tumors*. He also enjoys excellent health.

When I observed my control females developing tumors, I wondered why. The following subsections describe the possible causes I hypothesized.

The factors mentioned in the following paragraphs may have also caused my aspartame group rats to have more tumors than they would have had otherwise. For example, I gave my rats commercial rodent food, which I now believe may have contributed to both my control group and aspartame group tumors. If other animal studies feed their rats commercial rodent food, it may partially explain why their control groups developed tumors. A possible study would be to feed rats only organic food, give them pure water, and maintain them in an environment free of man-made chemicals, and compare the results with the control groups of other studies.

Pesticide-laden food

While thinking about possible causes of my control group tumors, I realized that the commercial grains I fed them probably had trace amounts of pesticides in them, and wondered if pesticides might cause tumors. I searched online for correlations between pesticides and cancer, and found the following substantiating information.

"In animal studies, many pesticides are carcinogenic, (e.g., organochlorines, creosote, and sulfallate) while others (notably, the organochlorines DDT, chlordane, and lindane) are tumor promoters."

According to researchers from Karolinska University Hospital in Stockholm, Sweden: *"In animal studies, many pesticides are carcinogenic, (e.g., organochlorines, creosote, and sulfallate) while others (notably, the organochlorines DDT, chlordane, and lindane) are tumor promoters. Some contaminants in commercial pesticide formulations also may pose a carcinogenic risk. In humans, arsenic compounds and insecticides used occupationally have been classified as carcinogens by the International Agency for Research on Cancer.... Organochlorine insecticides are linked with soft tissue sarcoma, non-Hodgkin's lymphoma (NHL), leukemia, and less consistently, with cancers of the lung and breast; and organophosphorous compounds are linked with NHL and leukemia."*[41]

In addition, organophosphate insecticides diazinon, dichlorvos, methyl parathion, and azamethiphos have been found to be genotoxic.[42] They alter the deoxyribonucleic acid (DNA) in living organisms, possibly causing mutations and cancer.[43] DNA contains instructions for creating and maintaining those organisms. It provides long-term information storage, similar to blueprints, recipes, or computer code. It allows your body to construct cell components, such as protein and the ribonucleic acid (RNA) used in protein synthesis and to carry genetic information for many viruses.[44] Damaged DNA passes from generation to generation. The pesticides you eat may affect your children, grandchildren, and their children.

From 4,000 to 20,000 cases of cancer per year are caused by permissible amounts of pesticides in food.

The National Academy of Sciences estimates that from 4,000 to 20,000 cases of cancer per year are caused by permissible amounts of pesticide residues in food.[45] It is likely that pesticides contributed to the tumors in both my control and aspartame-group females, since they ate the same food.

Note: In May 2009, researchers at the Moores Cancer Center at the University of California, San Diego, proposed a new model of cancer development. Epidemiologist Cedric Garland, Doctor of Public Health (DrPH), professor of family and preventive medicine at the UC San Diego School of Medicine, led the work. According to Garland, "The first event in cancer is loss of communication among cells due to, among other things, low vitamin D and calcium levels.... In this new model, we propose that this loss may play a key role in cancer by disrupting the communication between cells that is essential to healthy cell turnover, allowing more aggressive cancer cells to take over." Garland said that "previous theories linking vitamin D to certain cancers have been tested and confirmed in more than 200 epidemiological studies, and the understanding of its physiological basis stems from more than 2,500 laboratory studies."

The new model is called DINOMIT, where each letter stands for a different phase of cancer development. "The letter 'D' stands for disjunction, or loss of intercellular communication; 'I,' for initiation, where genetic mutations begin to play a role; 'N' for natural selection of the fastest-reproducing cancer cells; 'O' for overgrowth of cells; 'M' for metastasis, when cancer cells migrate to other tissues, where cancer can kill; 'I' refers to involution, and 'T' for transition, both dormant states that may occur in cancer and potentially be driven by replacing vitamin D." The currently accepted model states that genetic mutations are the earliest driving forces behind cancer.

Garland states that "Vitamin D may halt the first stage of the cancer process by re-establishing intercellular junctions in malignancies having an intact vitamin D receptor.... Vitamin D levels can be increased by modest supplementation with vitamin D3 in the range of 2000 IU/day."[46]

According to a UCSD broadcast, sufficient Vitamin D can also be attained by spending from 10 to 15 minutes a day in sunlight, with 40% of your skin exposed.

Herbicide-laden food

The European Union banned the use of the herbicide atrazine on food crops several years ago because of its association with birth defects, deformities, as well as breast and prostate cancer in humans. As the second most popular agricultural herbicide in the U.S., the EPA continues to allow the widespread use of atrazine on food crops, primarily to control weeds on corn and sugar cane. It is also used on residential lawns, and from there enters the ground water and waterways.[47]

Table 2-10 and Table 2-11 on page 2-18 show that the commercial rodent food I gave my rats contained rolled corn, ground corn, corn gluten meal, and cane molasses, all of which are likely to contain trace amounts of atrazine.

Due to its fat solubility, this chemical doesn't easily wash off from produce, and as a result, Americans consume large quantities each year by eating and drinking it. People living near commercial farms also breathe it into their bodies during crop dusting. After entering the body, it is stored in fat cells.[48]

During the past 10 years, scientists have noticed deformed genitalia and smaller voice boxes on frogs and other amphibians exposed to atrazine, making mating calls softer and reproduction impossible.

Atrazine has also been shown to interfere with the cellular uptake of dopamine. (See the discussion of dopamine and aggression on page 48 and "Does Aspartame Make You Fat?" on page 69.) The chemical also inhibits the mitochondrial ATP production of sperm, which then lacks the energy to swim through reproductive organs, resulting in infertility.[49] The herbicide also mimics the hormone estrogen. During the past 10 years, scientists have noticed deformed genitalia and smaller voice boxes on frogs and other amphibians exposed to atrazine, making their mating calls softer and reproduction impossible.

Atrazine was first introduced in 1958. In the late 1990s, scientists noticed increased fungal and viral diseases in exposed animals. Studies have confirmed that atrazine suppresses the immune system. Tiger salamanders exposed to atrazine are twice as likely to become infected with ambystoma tigrinum virus (ATV), causing internal hemorrhaging and death, as reported in *Ecological Applications*. When combined with the commonly-used fertilizer sodium nitrate, atrazine lowers the white blood cell count in salamanders by almost 20%. Amphibian skin is permeable, allowing toxins to be absorbed directly into the bloodstream, making them excellent indicators of environmental contamination.[50]

Research scientists from the Karolinska Institute in Stockholm, Sweden report that "*Epidemiologic studies ... have linked phenoxy acid herbicides or contaminants in them with soft tissue sarcoma and malignant lymphoma ... and triazine herbicides with ovarian cancer.*"[51]

Because my rats consumed corn and sugar cane products, it's probable that atrazine and other herbicides contributed to the tumors in both my aspartame and control groups.

GM food

Another possible cause of tumors in my control and aspartame groups may have been genetically modified (GM) grains in the commercial rodent food I gave them. In 2006, GM crops accounted for 61% of all corn planted in the U.S. and 89% of all soybeans.[52] Table 2-10 and Table 2-11 on page 2-18, show that the commercial rodent food I used included these ingredients: "*Rolled corn, ... ground corn, dehulled soybean meal ... corn gluten meal. ...*" It is therefore likely that my rats received both GM corn and soybeans.

The L-aspartic acid and L-phenylalanine in aspartame appear to be created using genetically engineered E. coli bacteria. E-coli is the most common species of fecal bacteria and is found only in human and animal excrement.

Note: The L-aspartic acid and L-phenylalanine in aspartame appear to be created using genetically engineered Escherichia coli (E. Coli) bacteria.[53] [54] [55] [56] E-coli is the most common species of fecal bacteria and is found only in human and animal excrement.[57]

This unsavory process is apparently used to maximize production output. A 1979 report of a Russian study published in Prikl Biokhim Mikrobiol found that E. Coli strain 85 synthesizes the largest amount of L-aspartic acid from fumarate and ammonium ions.[58] It is interesting to note that ammonium ions are created when ammonia, NH_3, accepts a proton, H^+.[59] One source of ammonia is decomposing urine and fecal matter.[60] Wouldn't it be efficient and cost effective if the E. Coli and ammonia used in aspartic acid production were both taken from the same source?

Even with the utmost care, an E. Coli synthesized chemical may contain traces of bacterial waste. A study reported in the January 2010 issue of the International Journal of Food Microbiology confirms this concern. Researchers from Hollins University in Virginia found E. Coli in soda and water samples from 30 different fast-food restaurants. Out of the 90 samples taken, 48% tested positive for coliform bacteria from human and animal feces, and 11% tested positive for E. Coli.[61]

According to anti-aspartame activist Betty Martini, Bill Deagle MD worked in a hospital near an aspartame plant in Georgia, and said the following about aspartame and genetic engineering: "While an E.R. doctor and primary care physician in Augusta, GA in 1987 and 1988, I was told a number of interesting facts about the adjacent aspartame factory. Bacteria with genes inserted generate a sludge which is centrifuged to remove the aspartame and many hundreds of contaminant organic and amino acids are present. We were told not to report illness or worker's compensation issues for fear of being fired by the hospital, now the Augusta Regional Medical Center. Many of their employees presented with psychiatric, neuropathy conditions, chronic fatigue and organic cases of loss of cognitive function."[62]

Aspartame also appears to damage the DNA of those consuming the sweetener, which means that all future generations may be adversely affected. A study at Cukurova University in Adana, Turkey, found that aspartame significantly damages chromosomes,[63] the threadlike strands of DNA and associated proteins that transmit hereditary information.[64]

The Trocho study in Spain found that aspartame damages DNA and may induce cell death and mutations. The damage is believed to be due to the formaldehyde that accumulates in the DNA after aspartame has broken down in the intestine.[65]

Unfortunately, it
appears that GM foods
were released into the
food chain without
sufficient knowledge
as to their long term
effects on our bodies
and food supply.

Unfortunately, it appears that GM foods were released into the food chain without sufficient knowledge as to their long term effects on our bodies and food supply. Take for example, what happened when genetically engineered L-tryptophan, a dietary supplement, was released in 1989. Before the FDA recalled it, the synthetic amino acid "*killed 37 Americans and permanently disabled or afflicted more than 5,000 others with a potentially fatal and painful blood disorder, eosinophilia myalgia syndrome (EMS).... The manufacturer, Showa Denko, Japan's third largest chemical company, had for the first time ... used GE bacteria to produce the over-the-counter supplement. It is believed that the bacteria somehow became contaminated during the recombinant DNA process. Showa Denko has already paid out over $2 billion in damages to EMS victims.*"[66]

In 1999, the British press revealed the research of Rowett Research Institute scientist Dr. Arpad Pusztai, who performed a rat study that found genetically engineered (GE) potatoes to be poisonous to mammals. The potatoes were spliced with DNA from the snowdrop plant and a viral promoter called the Cauliflower Mosaic Virus (CaMV).[67] The potatoes were found to damage the vital organs and immune systems of the rats. According to *Seeds of Deception* author Jeffrey Smith, "*Their white blood cells responded much more sluggishly than those fed a non-GM diet, leaving them more vulnerable to infection and disease. Organs related to the immune system, the thymus and spleen, showed some damage as well. Compared to rats fed a non-GM control diet, some of the GM fed rats had smaller, less developed brains, livers, and testicles. Other rats had enlarged tissues, including the pancreas and intestines. Some showed a partial atrophy of the liver. What's more, significant structural changes and a proliferation of cells in the stomach and intestines of GM-fed rats may have signaled an increased potential for cancer. The rats developed these serious health effects after only 10 days.*"[68]

Damage to the rats' stomach linings, apparently from a severe viral infection, was thought to have been caused by the CaMV promoter spliced into the potatoes and nearly all other GE crops in order to activate the foreign DNA.[69]

A Russian study conducted in 1998 confirmed the link between GM potatoes and cancer in lab rats, validating the research of Dr. Pusztai.[70]

Joseph Cummins, professor emeritus of genetics at the University of Western Ontario, considers the CaMV promoter to be the greatest threat from GE crops. He claims that "*The insertion of modified virus and insect virus genes into crops can create highly virulent new viruses.*" This is because over the eons, DNA has become a repository of genetic material, including now-dormant viruses. Cummins is concerned that the CaMV promoter may be activating such viruses. He is also concerned that the CaMV promoter may move between organisms, activating viruses whereever it goes. For example, the CaMV promoter in corn may move to DNA in the human stomach, and activate a dormant virus there. Cummins and others have warned that "*Horizontal transfer of the CaMV promoter ... has the potential to reactivate dormant viruses or create new viruses in all species to which it is transferred.*"[71]

This makes me wonder if the swine flu virus became dormant long ago, and was activated by the CaMV promoter in the GM corn shipped unlabeled from the U.S. to Mexico as part of the North American Free Trade Agreement (NAFTA). Since then, the corn has been planted illegally by Mexican farmers trying to compete with the heavier yields of American corn.[72]

I wonder if there might be unknown dormant monkey viruses inserted into the global population via vaccination, and if those dormant viruses are being activated by the CaMV promoter in GM foods.

I wonder if there might be unknown dormant monkey viruses inserted into the global population via vaccination programs, and if those dormant viruses are being activated by the CaMV promoter in GM foods.

For example, the live polio vaccine developed by Albert Sabin was given to about 100 million Americans between 1962 and 1965. Around 1957, however, Maurice Hilleman at Merck's vaccine division, discovered that the seed stock for the Sabin vaccine contained the activated cancer-causing simian virus 40 (SV40).[73] The virus had been injected into hamsters that subsequently grew tumors. While about 40 other simian viruses had been found and deactivated after being grown in contaminated monkey kidneys, it appears that SV40 may have remained active in some Sabin vaccines until the use of the vaccine was discontinued in 2000.[74] Dr. John Lednicky and Alfonso Cristaudo published a paper *"identifying SV40 gene sequences in childhood choroid plexus brain tumors and in mesotheliomas—rare cancers arising from cells lining the cavity surrounding the lung."*[75] So it appears that the virus has been involved in creating at least some human cancers. I would like to see studies searching for this virus in all human cancers.

According to author Leonard Horowitz DMD, *"Apparently, SV40 was not the only virus allowed to contaminate American-made vaccines. Using a combination of advanced tissue culture methods and genetic probes, Dr. John Martin, Professor of Pathology at the University of Southern California, assayed blood samples from patients with chronic fatigue syndrome and related nervous disorders. This work led to his discovery of unique cell-destroying viruses that were not recognized by the immune system. Termed 'stealth viruses,' the germs were able to cause persistent infections because they were missing specific genes which, if expressed, would evoke effective antiviral immunity. In March of 1995, Martin communicated to FDA officials that some stealth viruses clearly originated from African green monkey simian cytomegaloviruses—a type of herpes viruses that are known to infect man, monkeys, and other animals."* A 1972 study showed that *"simian cytomegalovirus was present in the kidney cultures of all eleven African green monkeys imported for vaccine production by Lederly—the sole producer of Orimune live polio vaccines for the United States."*[76]

In addition, according to Hilleman, *"There are genes that have to do with replication of cells, and if you activate them, screw them up in some way, or carry them from cell to cell, you can produce cancer."* The CaMV virus may activate such genes.[77] In May, 2009, the American Academy of Environmental Medicine (AAEM) implored *"Physicians to educate their patients, the medical community, and the public to avoid GM foods when possible and provide educational materials concerning GM foods and health risks."* They also called for labeling, long-term independent studies, and a moratorium on GM foods.[78] The organization's position paper mentioned the immune system problems, changes in major organs and gastrointestinal system publicized by Dr. Pusztai in 1999. It also described the health risks found in newer animal studies on GM foods, including infertility, accelerated aging, and insulin deregulation.[79]

Many doctors now prescribe GM-free diets. For example, Michigan internal medicine specialist Dr. Amy Dean says "*I strongly recommend patients eat strictly non-genetically modified foods.*" Dr. John Boyles, Ohio allergist states "*I used to test for soy allergies all the time, but now that soy is genetically engineered, it is so dangerous that I tell people never to eat it.*"

After reviewing over 600 scientific journals, world renowned biologist Pushpa M. Bhargava concluded that GM foods are major contributors to the deteriorating health of Americans.

After reviewing over 600 scientific journals, world renowned biologist Pushpa M. Bhargava concluded that GM foods are major contributors to the deteriorating health of Americans. Salk Institute biologist David Schubert warns that "*Children are the most likely to be adversely effected by toxins and other dietary problems*" from GM foods.[80]

According to author Jeffrey Smith in an online article published in May, 2009, "*After GM soy was fed to female rats, most of their babies died within three weeks, compared to a 10% death rate among the control group fed natural soy. The GM-fed babies were also smaller, and later had problems getting pregnant. When male rats were fed GM soy, their testicles actually changed from their normal pink to dark blue. Mice fed GM soy had altered sperm. Even the embryos of GM fed parent mice had significant changes in their DNA. Mice fed GM corn in an Austrian government study had fewer babies, which were also smaller than normal.*"[81]

Buffalo eating GM cottonseed in India had prolapsed uteruses, infertility, spontaneous abortions, premature births, and many calves died. Around two dozen U.S. farmers claimed that thousands of pigs became sterile from eating GM corn. Some had false pregnancies, even giving birth to bags of water. When eating the same corn, cows and bulls also became infertile.[82]

Biotech companies engineer GM corn and cotton to produce a pesticide in each cell from a soil bacterium similar to Bacillus anthrax,[83] called bacillus thuringiensis (Bt) toxin. Insects biting the plants die when the poison splits open their stomachs.[84]

When sheep grazed on Bt-cotton plants after a harvest in India, thousands of them died. "*Investigators said preliminary evidence 'strongly suggests that the sheep mortality was due to a toxin. ... most probably Bt-toxin.'*" When the Deccan Development Society did a follow-up study, all sheep eating Bt-cotton plants were dead within a month, while those eating natural cotton stayed healthy. In Andhra Pradesh, 13 buffalo died after three days of grazing on Bt-cotton plants. Bt-corn was implicated in the deaths of chickens, horses and water buffaloes in The Philippines, and cows in Germany.[85]

In lab studies, twice as many chickens fed GM corn died in one lab study. In a study of 20 rats eating GM tomatoes, seven developed bleeding stomachs, and seven others died within 14 days.[86]

Only one human study has been published, and reveals possibly the most problematic issue of GM foods. Genes spliced into GM soybeans enter the DNA of bacteria inside the human intestine and continue to be activated. So even if we no longer eat GM foods, the potentially harmful proteins continue to be produced within us.

Only one human study has been published. It reveals possibly the most problematic issue of GM foods. Genes spliced into GM soybeans enter the DNA of bacteria inside the human intestine and continue to be activated. So even if we no longer eat GM food, the potentially harmful proteins continue to be produced within us. So for example, if you eat Bt-corn, the intestinal bacteria to which the Bt-gene is transferred may continue to produce and distribute the Bt-pesticide within your body for the rest of your life.[87]

Once a GM crop is released into the environment, it can cross pollinate with non-GM crops. Yet according to famed Canadian geneticist David Suzuki, "*The* [safety] *experiments simply haven't been done and we now have become the guinea pigs.*" He adds, "*Anyone that says, 'Oh, we know that this is perfectly safe,' I say is either unbelievably stupid or deliberately lying.*"[88]

If GM foods cause cancer, heart disease, reproductive problems, autism, obesity, diabetes, asthma, or allergies, we may never know it. Animals eating GM foods have had a wide range of problems. However, within nine years of introducing GM crops on a large scale in 1996, the percentage of the population suffering from three or more chronic diseases went from 7% to 13%.[89]

To avoid GM foods, eat organic or "*non-GMO*." A downloadable *Non-GMO Shopping Guide* in pocket form is available from the Institute for Responsible Technology and the Center for Food Safety at http://www.responsibletechnology.org/DocumentFiles/144.pdf. It can also be found in natural food stores and many doctors' offices. If even a small percentage of the population chooses to eat non-GM food, the food industry may respond as happened in Europe, and remove all GM ingredients.[90]

By current U.S. law, organic foods cannot contain GM components, but some predict that within 10 years, it will be impossible not to eat GM food. So we'll likely be subject to more genetically engineered disasters, like the killer queen bees that were accidentally released into the Western Hemisphere in 1957. Brazilian geneticists were hoping to boost crop pollination and production by crossbreeding African bees with honey bees from Europe to create a gentle but super-productive strain.[91]

African bee stings are no more potent than those of ordinary bees, but the bees are far more aggressive and attack in swarms. For example, someone disturbing a killer hive would be stung at least 200 times, whereas a similar disturbance of a European bee hive might result in a couple dozen stings. Now African bees are displacing more fragile honey bees, forming an average of 16 new hives per year, while European bees form only two to three.[92] Many of those are dying out in record numbers as part of a phenomenon called *colony collapse disorder*. Some blame Bt-engineered plants with built in pesticides.[93] The Bt-toxin is present in the pollen of such plants, since it is generated in all parts of the plants. The bees use pollen to create honey, which is probably toxic to them, since it appears to kill much larger mammals as described earlier.

Genetic studies by Deborah Smith at the University of Michigan, and Glenn Hall at the University of Florida, have demonstrated that the cross-bred bees of the Brazilian experiment have died off, and those spreading throughout the Americas are now pure African bees.[94]

The question is, will our bodies be able adapt to the strange new varieties of GM food and other Frankenstein-style creations that will soon be dominating our landscape? Or will cancer and more new diseases like the swine flu, avian flu, and SARS take over our lives and threaten our long-term survival? Clearly, we should take a lesson from the animals. Smith's book provides multiple examples where geese, cows, hogs, squirrels, elk, deer, raccoons, mice, and rats were given the choice of eating GM or non-GM grains. In each case, they avoided GM grains and ate freely from non-GM grains.[95]

The GM grains I fed my rats may have affected their immune systems, making them more susceptible to tumors and other adverse effects.

Other toxins in commercial rodent food

As shown in Table 2-10 and Table 2-11 on page 2-18, the food I fed my rats included soy, animal and fish meals.

Soy

Soy has been touted as a high protein food with many health benefits. However, I have been avoiding it since 2004 due to adverse effects I personally experienced. For instance, I had post-menopausal bleeding that I believe was brought on by the phytoestrogens in soy,[96] and the many hormones—including several estrogens—in dairy.[97] I had read that 20% of women with such bleeding suffer from uterine cancer, and I had a friend who recently died from that disease. When I quit eating soy and dairy, the bleeding disappeared.

Recall the discussion in "Possible non-inert components of NutraSweet" on page 95, where glutamate, also referred to as glutamic acid, has been found in elevated levels in the blood of cancer and AIDS patients. According to the *Phytochemical and Ethnobotanical Database* website provided by the USDA, soybeans contain between 70,680 and 77,280 ppm of glutamic acid, comprising almost 10% of the bean.[98]

I have not found evidence that soy causes uterine cancer, however a 2002 Singapore health study reported that soy appears to increase the risk of bladder cancer.[99]

The phytoestrogens from soy may also cause lung cancer. According to University of Pittsburgh research findings presented in April 2000, *"Estrogen, long known for its role in fueling the growth of breast cancer, may spur the same insidious process in lung cancer. ... The results are the first to directly demonstrate increased growth of non-small cell lung cancer in the presence of estrogen."*[100]

In December 2002, the National Institute of Environmental Health Sciences added estrogen to its list of known cancer-causing agents. According to a 2003 article from Columbia University, *"For years, estrogen has been a suspected carcinogen, since strong epidemiological evidence associates the hormone to breast, endometrial, and uterine cancers. Women who begin menstruating early, or who start menopause late, produce more estrogen over their lifetimes and have a higher risk of breast cancer."*[101]

In December 2002, the National Institute of Environmental Health Sciences added estrogen to its list of known cancer-causing agents.

In 2007, the Cancer Council of New South Wales, Australia, issued guidelines "*warning about the dangers of high-soy diets and soy supplements for cancer patients and those people in remission from cancer. At particular risk are people suffering from hormone-dependent cancers, including breast and prostate cancer—the two most common types of cancer in Australia.*"[102]

It's therefore possible that soy contributed to the tumors of both my aspartame and control group rats.

Meat and poultry meals

The food I gave my rats also included meat and poultry meal. Howard Lyman, author of *Mad Cowboy: Plain Truth from the Cattle Rancher who won't Eat Meat*, was sued by members of the beef industry along with Oprah Winfrey after statements they made on her show. (The beef industry lost the lawsuit.) Lyman's book colorfully describes the origins of meat meal:

"There is simply no such thing in America as an animal too ravaged by disease, too cancerous, or too putrid to be welcomed by the all-embracing arms of the renderer."

"When a cow is slaughtered, about half of it by weight is not eaten by humans: the intestines and their contents, the head, hooves, and horns, as well as bones and blood. These are dumped into giant grinders at rendering plants, as are the entire bodies of cows and other farm animals known to be diseased. Rendering is a $2.4-billion-a-year industry, processing forty billion pounds of dead animals a year. There is simply no such thing in America as an animal too ravaged by disease, too cancerous, or too putrid to be welcomed by the all-embracing arms of the renderer. Another staple of the renderer's diet, in addition to farm animals, is euthanized pets—the six or seven million dogs and cats that are killed in animal shelters every year. ... Added to the blend are the euthanized catch of animal control agencies, and roadkill. (Roadkill is not collected daily, and in the summer, the better roadkill collection crews can generally smell it before they can see it.) When this gruesome mix is ground and steam-cooked ... the heavier protein material is dried and pulverized into a brown powder—about a quarter of which consists of fecal material. The powder is used as an additive to almost all pet food as well as to livestock feed. ... In 1995, five million tons of processed slaughterhouse leftovers were sold for animal feed in the United States."[103]

As inflammatory and unimaginable as Lyman's description sounds, fecal matter is taken very seriously by the animal-feed industry. It's use is defended in an online article discussing the relevant safety concerns, including "*its high bacteriological activity, the accumulation of anti-metabolites, drugs and other non-nutritional excretory products partly derived from the ration.*[104]

The article describes concerns about the excessive accumulation of heavy metals, including lead, mercury, and cadmium; the accumulation of medicinal drugs such as antibiotics, coccidiostatics, and sulfa drugs; and the accumulation of "*insecticides, herbicides, wood preservatives, mycotoxins and hormones.*" It also addresses concerns about the "*harmful organisms transmittable via wastes to other animals and to man.*"[105]

The article appears to defend the use of fecal matter as animal feed by stating: "*These problems, however, do not relate to wastes alone: conventional feeds may contain a large number of contaminants in the form of phytotoxins, pesticides, pathogens and other xenobiotics.*"[106] It appears to be reiterating some of the points I made earlier about commercial rodent food and it's possible causes of adverse effects on my rats.

The article then addresses each of these concerns in detail, citing studies that show that relatively few problems exist from adding fecal matter to animal feed. The article states that *"Over two decades of experimental and field observations have so far produced no scientific evidence to show that animal-waste recycling poses any health risks provided the waste is properly processed and the ration carefully balanced."*[107]

My skepticism regarding this conclusion is two fold. First, due to the complex interactions and the possible deterioration of the level of health of the animals from each factor, the accumulation of negative effects from all factors may be far greater than the sum of the individual and negligible adverse effects. This was shown using only four chemicals as described in "Chemical cocktails multiply toxic effects" on page 99. It would be interesting to multiply the number of chemicals studied to more closely simulate the quantity we're consuming in our real-world food, water, and air supply.

The other issue is the length of time the studies were undertaken. For example, the article describes a 1978 toxicological research study in which steers were fed dried manure as 30% of their diet for 180 days, or approximately six months. That study *"found that all physiological parameters (blood, urine, serum indicator enzymes, pathological examination of tissues, microsomal mixed-function oxidase activities in post mortem liver) were normal."*[108] Yet the average life expectancy of a steer is around 15 years.[109] So that study was continued for only (six months)/(15 years) = (0.5 years)/(15 years) = 0.03 = 3% of the lifetime of an average steer. Therefore we really don't know the long term toxicological effects on a steer eating such a large amount of fecal matter.

> One factor of significance to my experiment is the high levels of hormones found in animal feces.

One factor of significance to my experiment is the high level of hormones found in animal feces. In a 1942 experiment on chicks, precocious comb and wattle growth were found when dried fecal matter from cows was incorporated into their diet. Subsequent studies found the development of testicles and ovaries to be retarded when chicks were fed dried cow feces. Estrogens were found in livestock waste in 1957. Lambs fed 1 mg of the synthetic estrogen diethylstilbestrol (DES) per day excreted 76% of the daily dose, and those fed 2 mg excreted 84% of the dose. This means that 24% of the 1 mg dose and 16% of the 2 mg dose remained in their bodies. A 1968 study found an increase in the rate of estrogen in the fecal matter of a cow during her first seven months of pregnancy, and a 1969 experiment found measurable amounts of estrone and estradiol in the manure of layer hens. Androgenic and estrogenic activity were reported in poultry manure in 1978. Sexual hormones in pig waste were reported in 1977.[110]

Recall that in 2002, estrogen was added to the list of carcinogens by the National Institute of Environmental Health Sciences. (See "Soy" in "Other toxins in commercial rodent food" on page 108.) The estrogen from the fecal matter in the meat and poultry meals of the rodent food I fed my rats may therefore have contributed to the tumors in both my experimental and control groups. (See Table 2-10 and Table 2-11 on page 2-18.)

In addition, meat and poultry meals are made from animals that probably consumed GM corn and other GM foods, which may also have contributed to the tumors in both my experimental and control groups. (See "GM food" on page 102.)

Finally, the animal protein in the meat and poultry meals may itself have contributed to the tumors in both my aspartame and control groups. T. Colin Campbell, PhD directed the China Study, called the *"Grand Prix of Epidemiology"* by *The New York Times*. The project is considered *"the most comprehensive study of diet, lifestyle and disease ever done with humans in the history of biomedical research."* Performed by researchers at Cornell University, Oxford University and the Chinese Academy of Preventive Medicine, its participants surveyed a wide range of diseases, diet, and lifestyle factors in 2,400 counties of rural China and Taiwan. Beginning in 1983 and still ongoing in 2006, the project has resulted in over *"8,000 statistically significant associations between various dietary factors and disease!"*[111]

> *"People who ate the most animal-based foods got the most chronic disease. Even relatively small intakes of animal-based food were associated with adverse effects. People who ate the most plant-based foods were the healthiest and tended to avoid chronic disease."*

The most significant finding of the study is the correlation between the consumption of animal-based foods and disease. According to the report: *"People who ate the most animal-based foods got the most chronic disease. Even relatively small intakes of animal-based food were associated with adverse effects. People who ate the most plant-based foods were the healthiest and tended to avoid chronic disease."*[112]

Regarding the relationship between cancer and diet, Campbell says *"Published data show that animal protein promotes the growth of tumors. Animal protein increases the levels of a hormone, [insulin-like growth factor] IGF-1, which is a risk factor for cancer, and high-casein (the main protein of cow's milk) diets allow more carcinogens into cells, which allow more dangerous carcinogen products to bind to DNA, which allow more mutagenic reactions that give rise to cancer cells, which allow more rapid growth of tumors once they are initially formed. ... We now have a deep and broad range of evidence showing that a whole foods, plant-based diet is best for cancer."*[113]

Campbell also supervised numerous animal studies confirming these findings. Astoundingly, he reports that *"Low-protein diets inhibited the initiation of cancer by [the highly carcinogenic chemical] aflatoxin, regardless of how much of this carcinogen was administered to these animals. After cancer initiation was completed, low-protein diets also dramatically blocked subsequent cancer growth.... In fact, dietary protein proved to be so powerful in its effect that we could turn on and turn off cancer growth simply by changing the level consumed."*[114]

I personally find the statement about the main protein in cow's milk, casein, to be very interesting. In April 2009, I felt what I believe was a growth in the lymph gland of my left armpit. When I ate dairy, the growth became painful and felt enlarged. When I abstained, the pain went away and the growth became imperceptible. Needless to say, that experience inspired me to stay away from dairy. It was especially scary because a friend passed on from lymphoma in May 2008. It started as a tumor in his armpit that grew to the size of an orange or small grapefruit, and he eventually had about 20 tumors throughout his torso. I noticed that he ate dairy from time to time, though most of the time, he ate an incredibly healthy diet. He also loved Asian food, which is usually loaded with glutamic acid, due to the wide-spread use of soy products. As mentioned earlier, studies have shown that cancer and AIDs patients have elevated glutamic acid levels. See the discussion of "Soy" in "Other toxins in commercial rodent food" on page 108.

The China Study also supports the recent UCSD research regarding vitamin D and cancer introduced on page 101. According to Campbell, *"Increased intakes of animal protein ... enhance the production of insulin-like growth factor IGF-1 and this enhances cancer cell growth. ... When blood levels of* [vitamin D] *are depressed, IGF-1 simultaneously becomes more active. Together these factors increase the birth of new cells while simultaneously inhibiting the removal of old cells, both favoring the development of cancer."*[115]

Fish meal

It appears that the fish meal in the food I fed my rats may have also contributed to the tumors of both my aspartame and control groups.

In an online article, David Biello reports that *"many streams, rivers and lakes already bear warning signs that the fish caught within them may contain dangerously high levels of mercury, which can cause brain damage. But, according to a new study, these fish may also be carrying enough chemicals that mimic the female hormone estrogen to cause breast cancer cells to grow."*[116]

Conrad Volz is co-director of exposure assessment at the University of Pittsburgh Cancer Institute's Center for Environmental Ecology. He and his colleagues examined extracts from 21 catfish and six white bass that were caught in the rivers around Pittsburgh. They also studied several store-bought fish as controls.

"Using an organic solvent, the researchers created an extract from the skin, flesh and fat of the various fish. They then bathed a breast cancer cell line ... in the extract." The cell line was used because it has estrogen receptors, so that if estrogens are present, the cell line will proliferate. The extracts from two white bass and five catfish caused the breast cancer cells to thrive. *"The highest response came from fish caught in the industrial section of the Monongahela River, the site of steel production for over 100 years. The broadest response was from the sewer outflows of the sewage treatment plants, where extracts from three of the four catfish caught there caused the breast cancer cells to grow."* According to Volz, *"Sewage might be more responsible for putting estrogenic chemicals in the water than the industries alone. All of the hormone replacement products that women use go down the drain, along with birth control pills, antibacterial soaps, and many of the plastics we use, like Bisphenol A, have such effects."* Recall that estrogen is a carcinogen, as discussed in "Soy" on page 108.

In addition to the carcinogenic effects of the estrogens, the genders of nine fish were indeterminate. Volze says that *"Increased estrogenic active substances in the water are changing males so that they are indistinguishable from females."* The study found eggs in the gonads of some males, and some secreted a yolk sac protein—functions normally limited to females.

"Many streams, rivers and lakes already bear warning signs that the fish caught within them may contain dangerously high levels of mercury, which can cause brain damage. But, according to a new study, these fish may also be carrying enough chemicals that mimic the female hormone estrogen to cause breast cancer cells to grow."

Store-bought bass from Lake Erie also caused proliferation of the breast cancer cells. In addition, it contained higher levels of mercury, arsenic and other contaminants. *"These fish, again, were in waters that were seeing industrial waste as well as possible combined sewer outflows,"* Volz states, *"This isn't just happening in Pittsburgh, this is happening everywhere in the industrialized world."*

Use of plastic water bottles

Another factor I thought might have caused my experimental and control rats to develop tumors is the plastic bottles I used for their water. In recent years, much research has surfaced about plastics leaching into the drinking water from plastic bottles, especially those exposed to heat. Some of my rat cages were on a southern-facing wall, and some of the water bottles of the controls, in particular, were exposed to direct sunlight, which would have heated their water bottles. I'm not sure if the bottles I used were safe because there is so much conflicting information. But I'm including this discussion because I feel it is important.

One of the plastic compounds that can be released from plastics is bisphenol A (BPA), a building block of several important plastics, such as polycarbonates.[117] BPA is found in baby bottles, food and beverage containers, linings of metal food cans, dental sealants and many other products. It's also in the air, dust, rivers and estuaries—and Americans of all ages, including newborns. Over 2 billion pounds of BPA are produced in the U.S. each year. Over 6 billion pounds are produced worldwide, generating an estimated $1 million a day for corporations such as Bayer, Dow, GE Plastics and Sunoco.[118]

BPA is an endocrine disrupter. Low doses can mimic the body's own hormones. It was first suspected of being hazardous to humans when evidence of its estrogenicity was found in rat experiments conducted in the 1930s.

BPA is an endocrine disrupter. Low doses can mimic the body's own hormones. It was first suspected of being hazardous to humans when evidence of its estrogenicity was found in rat experiments conducted in the 1930s. However, the adverse effects from low-dose exposure on laboratory animals were not reported until 1997. Since then, more than 100 studies stating health concerns have been published about the chemical.[119]

Those with greatest sensitivity to the chemical appear to be the young. BPA has been found to be carcinogenic and possibly neurotoxic at low doses in animals. It's also been suggested to be linked to obesity.[120] An experiment comparing the effects of the estrogen 17β-estradiol (E2) to those of BPA finds *"The exposure of adult mice to a single low dose (10 μg/kg) of either E2 or BPA induces a rapid decrease in glycemia that correlates with a rise of plasma insulin.... After four days of treatment with E2 or BPA, these mice developed chronic hyperinsulinemia, and their glucose and insulin tolerance tests were altered."*[121] Such physiological effects have been associated with weight gain and obesity.[122] What's more, these experiments show the link between environmental estrogens and insulin resistance, increasing the risk of developing type 2 diabetes mellitus, hypertension, and dyslipidemia, a disruption of the lipids (the fats) in the blood.[123]

A study by the Yale School of Medicine showed that *"adverse neurological effects occur in non-human primates regularly exposed to bisphenol A at levels equal to the United States Environmental Protection Agency's (EPA) maximum safe dose of 50 µg/kg/day."* The study also *"found a connection between BPA and interference with brain cell connections vital to memory, learning and mood."*[124]

A consensus statement in 2007, by 38 international experts concluded: *"The wide range of adverse effects of low doses of BPA in laboratory animals exposed both during development and in adulthood is a great cause for concern with regard to the potential for similar adverse effects in humans. Recent trends in human diseases relate to adverse effects observed in experimental animals exposed to low doses of BPA:*

- *Increase in breast and prostate cancer*
- *Uro-genital abnormalities in male babies*
- *Decline in semen quality in men*
- *Early onset of puberty in girls*
- *Metabolic disorders including insulin-resistant (type 2) diabetes*
- *Obesity in children and adults*
- *Neurobehavioral problems such as ADHD"*[125]

A panel convened by the U.S. National Institutes of Health and a 2008 report by the U.S. National Toxicology Program (NTP) agreed that there is concern about the *"effects on the brain, behavior, and prostate gland in fetuses, infants, and children at current human exposures to bisphenol A."* [126]

"BPA can affect the hearts of women, can permanently damage the DNA of mice, and appear to be pouring into the human body from a variety of unknown sources."

New research was reported at an Endocrine Society meeting in 2009. Troubling data was presented showing *"BPA can affect the hearts of women, can permanently damage the DNA of mice, and appear to be pouring into the human body from a variety of unknown sources."*[127]

To reduce your exposure to BPA:

- Minimize the use of plastics, plastic wraps and containers.
- Use glass baby bottles and dishes.
- Discard old, scratched plastic dishes and containers. Don't wash plastic dishes in the dishwasher using strong detergents.
- Avoid canned foods and drinks. They are lined with plastic.

Why was my control group relatively healthy?

When a preliminary version of this report was summarized and leaked on the Internet without my permission, it caused a stir on blogs reddit.com and digg.com. One blogger commented that my control group was too healthy compared to those from other studies. The person claimed that I must have faked my data. As mentioned earlier, that comment inspired me to write this appendix.

I had actually been concerned when rats from my control group developed tumors, but the blogger made me think of reasons my control group might have been relatively healthy, as described in the following subsections.

Drinking well water

When my control rats started developing tumors, I thought the well water I was giving them might be polluted, as is the water in many U.S. wells. It can become contaminated by pesticide and herbicide runoffs and other toxic chemicals, such as MTBE—the gasoline additive found carcinogenic by Dr. Soffritti as discussed on page 14. Our neighbor across the street had his well water tested, however, and it was free of contaminants. Since we tap into the same underground source, I assume that our water is also pure. Tap water is generally not so pure, however, and if it is used in laboratories, that may help explain why my control group was healthier than most.

Chemical compounds in tap water

Between 2006 and 2007, the Southern Nevada Water Authority in Las Vegas Nevada analyzed the tap water from 19 U.S. water utilities looking for 51 chemical compounds. The study found the widespread low-level presence of pharmaceuticals and hormonally active chemicals. The 11 most frequently detected compounds were:

- Atenolol, a beta-blocker for cardiovascular disease

- Atrazine, an herbicide implicated in the decline of fish stocks and changes in animal behavior. (For a discussion of Atrazine, see "Herbicide-laden food" on page 101.)

- Carbamazepine, a mood-stabilizing drug for bipolar disorder

- Estrone, an estrogen blamed for gender-bending changes in fish

- Gemfibrozil, an anti-cholesterol drug

- Meprobamate, a tranquilizer

- Naproxen, a painkiller and anti-inflammatory drug

- Phenytoin, an anticonvulsant for treating epilepsy

- Sulfamethoxazole, an antibiotic

- TCEP, a reducing agent used in molecular biology

- Trimethoprim, an antibiotic[128]

Estrogens in tap water

Note that estrone, an estrogen, was listed in the previous subsection. A number of years ago, a water quality scientist from San Diego State University spoke on KPBS public radio in San Diego. He said that there are thousands of trace chemicals in our public drinking water, and many mimic estrogen.

In a 2007 article, researchers from the University of Pittsburgh reported that *"Most pharmaceutical estrogens and xenoestrogens are introduced into the environment through municipal waste water treatment plant (WWTP) effluent sources. These effluents contain synthetic compounds; surfactants, flame retardants and halogenated hydrocarbons that can mimic estrogens; and are discharged directly into rivers and lakes. As rivers and lakes are used for water and food supply and recreation, and wastewater effluent usage*

> Between 2006 and 2007, the Southern Nevada Water Authority in Las Vegas analyzed the tap water from 19 U.S. water utilities looking for 51 chemical compounds. The study found the widespread low-level presence of pharmaceuticals and hormonally active chemicals.

increases, the presence and concentration of xenoestrogens in surface water becomes a valid public health concern. Additionally, many USA cities have significant combined sewer overflows releasing untreated sewage directly into surface waters, thus increasing the amounts of xenoestrogens finding their way into drinking water supplies and commercial and subsistence fishing habitat.

"In the United States, humans are exposed daily to both pharmaceutical and xenoestrogens which have been implicated in various human health outcomes, such as testicular dysgenesis syndrome including testicular cancer and breast cancer in women. Also, they can have adverse reproductive effects in aquatic wildlife through sex reversals, production of intersex individuals, alterations in mating, and prevention of gonadal maturation.... Each xenoestrogen exhibits its own wildlife or human health risk, but synergistic effects could occur with xenoestrogen mixtures."[129]

As mentioned in "Soy" on page 108, in 2002 estrogen was declared carcinogenic by the National Institute of Environmental Health Sciences in 2002. So it's possible that studies using tap water may have more tumors in their control groups due to chemicals in the water administered to their subjects.

Disinfection by products in tap water

Another threat from tap water consists of the chemicals used to disinfect it and more critically, their disinfection by products (DBPs).

Another threat from tap water consists of the chemicals used to disinfect it and more critically, their disinfection by products (DBPs). According to researcher Robert Slovak, a pioneer in water filtration, DBPs, rather than chlorine, are responsible for the most toxic effects of chlorinated water. Slovak claims that DBPs are over 10,000 times more toxic than chlorine. He believes that DPBs are worse than all other toxins in tap water, including fluoride and pharmaceutical drugs.[130]

Most disinfection methods used by water treatment facilities use chlorine, chlorine dioxide, and chloramines to kill disease-causing microorganisms. Toxic chemical by products are created, however, when such disinfectants react with organic matter like decaying vegetation. The following disinfectant by products are most commonly formed when chlorine is used:

- Trihalomethanes (THMs)

- Haloacetic acids (HAAs)[131]

THMs have been found to cause cancer in laboratory animals. DBPs have also been linked to reproductive problems in animals and humans. Lifetime consumption of chlorine-treated water has been found to more than double the risk of bladder and rectal cancers for some risk groups. For example, one study reports that smoking men who drank chlorinated tap water for over 40 years faced double the risk of bladder cancer compared with smoking men who drank non-chlorinated water.[132]

Another study found rates for rectal cancers for both males and females correlated with the length of time chlorinated water has been consumed. Those on low-fiber diets who drank chlorinated water for 40 years or more increased their risk for rectal cancer by more than two-fold, compared with those drinking non-chlorinated water.[133]

DBPs may be even more dangerous when absorbed through the skin. The *Journal of Environmental Sciences* reported a study that found swimming in a chlorinated pool to be a cancer risk from THMs. The report specified the following order of THM cancer risk:

- Skin exposure from swimming
- Gastro-intestinal exposure from tap water
- Skin exposure from tap water
- Gastro-intestinal exposure from swimming[134]

The risk of cancer from skin exposure while swimming in a chlorinated pool was more than 94% of the total risk resulting from THM exposure.

The risk of cancer from skin exposure while swimming in a chlorinated pool was more than 94% of the total risk resulting from THM exposure. THMs in chlorinated pools are also linked with stillbirths, spontaneous abortions, and congenital malformations. While reverse osmosis filters are efficient at filtering out DPBs, Slovak says that some water filtration systems are incapable of filtering them out, and there is currently no point-of-entry, entire-house water filtration system certified to filter them out.[135]

Fluoride in tap water

Many states and cities in the U.S. and other countries are currently fluoridating their drinking water with the purpose of reducing dental cavities in those drinking the water. Numerous studies, however, have shown fluoridation increasing the risk of various types of cancers. For example, a 1975 study regarding fluoridation and cancer was conducted by Dr. Dean Burk, former chief chemist of the National Cancer Institute, and Dr. John Yiamouyiannis. The study compared the number of deaths from cancer per year in fluoridated versus non-fluoridated areas. The 10 largest fluoridated cities were compared against the 10 largest non-fluoridated cities. After 13 to 17 years, cities fluoridating their tap water had a 10 percent increase in cancer death rates compared to their non-fluoridated counterparts. The study was repeated by the Centers for Disease Control and Prevention (CDC) using a greater number of cities with similar results. Other studies have been even more alarming. Dr. Donald Austin of the California Tumor Registry found cancer death rates were 40% higher in fluoridated California communities. In fluoridated Canadian cities, Dr. Victor Cecilioni found cancer death rates to be 15 to 25% higher than those in non-fluoridated cities.[136]

The U.S. Congress ordered a study conducted by the Battelle Memorial Institute in Columbus, Ohio. In February 1989, the study reported that a 45 ppm solution of fluoride resulted in a 12% increase in cancers of the tongue, gums and other oral cancers. Subsequent studies showed the incidence of oral cancers was from 33% to 50% greater in fluoridated versus non-fluoridated cities.[137] The longer you drink fluoridated water, the Battelle study reported, the higher your bone fluoride levels. Animals exposed to a 45 ppm mixture of fluoridated drinking water reportedly had an increased risk of a rare bone cancer called osteosarcoma. Fluoride concentrations in bones during human studies were found at levels of more than 2,000 ppm. Reports from the National Cancer Institute and a 1992 study by the New Jersey Department of Health found increases of up to 50% of osteosarcoma in young men drinking fluoridated water.

The New Jersey study reported a 3 to 7 times greater incidence of osteosarcoma in young men in fluoridated communities.[138]

Proctor & Gamble scientists found a link between fluoride ingestion and bone cancer risk before adding fluoride to Crest toothpaste.

Proctor & Gamble scientists found a link between fluoride ingestion and bone cancer risk before adding fluoride to Crest toothpaste. They found genetic damage to cells exposed to 1 ppm fluoride, the dose added to municipal drinking water. The correlation to genetic damage has been confirmed by other researchers. Other types of cancers correlated with fluoride include:

- A 35 percent increase in lung cancer from industrial exposure to airborne fluoride

- A 129 percent increase in laryngeal cancer

- An 84 percent increase in bladder cancer

- A rare liver tumor also produced in experimental animals by uranium[139]

Neurosurgeon Dr. Russell Blaylock warns that fluoride may also be linked to neurological impairment, brain diseases like Alzheimer's, male impotence and infertility, sleep impairment, retardation in children, and numerous cancers. He recommends that we avoid:

- Fluoridated water

- Teas high in fluoride. (See the discussion of tea starting on page page 96).

- Toothpaste with fluoride. (Health food stores offer fluoride-free toothpaste.)

- Vaccinations containing fluoride and aluminum

- Pesticides and herbicides

- Medications containing fluoride

- California wines

- Soy products, as they are high in fluoride, glutamic acid, aluminum, and manganese, all known neurotoxins. (He recommends that mothers avoid giving their children soy-based infant formulas, especially if reconstituted with fluoridated water. The baby brain is most vulnerable to these brain toxins.)[140]

Laboratories using fluoridated tap water in their experiments may therefore have increased cancer rates in both their experimental and control animals. I gave my rats well water, which may explain why my controls were healthier than those in other studies.

Getting fresh air

Due to a lack of indoor space, I kept my rats outside where they received pure mountain air. I believe that this may have contributed to their overall health when compared to rats maintained indoors, due to indoor air pollution. Have you ever noticed the strong smells inside a hospital? That's how I imagine most test laboratories smell as well. I was unable to find articles about the air quality inside test labs, but I would assume that it is more polluted with chemicals than most home environments.

A San Francisco Chronicle article in May 2004 states that *"Frying chicken at the stove, spraying ants with insecticide, taking a hot shower, plugging in a room freshener, or sudsing the rug with detergent—all these release chemicals that swirl around rooms like invisible dust devils. Household products, furnishings and cosmetics release vapors and particles that people can inhale or absorb through the skin. Then there are the pollutants that are tracked into the house from outside or allowed to waft through open windows that add to the hazard. Plunking down on a sofa, vacuuming the rug or making the bed stirs up the chemical-laden dust...."*[141]

Researchers on indoor air pollution are warning that levels of pollution in houses are several times higher than outdoor pollution, even that of highly polluted cities.

Researchers on indoor air pollution are warning that levels of pollution in houses are several times higher than outdoor pollution, even that of highly polluted cities. Radon gas, tobacco smoke, mold, lead particles, some pesticides and asbestos have been found to be potential contributors to respiratory diseases, cancer, and other diseases. Chemicals now thought to be potential hazards include those in flame retardants, plastic softeners, and surfactants in cosmetics and detergents.[142]

In 2004, 2,500 people who didn't work with chemicals were tested by the Mount Sinai School of Medicine for more than 200 industrial chemicals. A total of 167 chemicals were found in their bodies, averaging 91 chemicals per person. Of those, 55 cause cancer, and the rest are linked to health problems of the reproductive, cardiovascular, nervous, and immune systems.[143]

According to an article about the study *"The Toxic Substances Control Act doesn't require that the U.S. Environmental Protection Agency ask for toxicology tests on many thousands of chemicals on the market. In addition, each year the EPA receives applications for 2,000 new chemicals—or six a day. Yet, under the law, the agency can't require studies from the manufacturers proving that the chemicals are safe for humans and the environment unless the agency can show that the chemical poses a significant risk."*[144]

A study published in *Environmental Science & Technology* in 2003 discovered 90 chemicals in the air and dust of 120 houses in Cape Cod Massachusetts. They included chemicals that cause neurological problems, cancer, birth defects, and that disrupt the endocrine system by mimicking and increasing estrogen in lab animals. More than 20 chemicals were found in each house, including banned substances such as DDT and PCBs.[145]

Again, we see that estrogen may play a role in the development of tumors, this time from indoor air pollution. However, my rats were not exposed to such pollutants, and perhaps that is one reason why my control rats may have been healthier than those in other laboratory studies.

Notes

G

For More Info

The resources listed in this appendix provide reference information for the topics described throughout this report.

Websites, videos, audios, books, and support groups

For links to support groups, websites, videos, audios, and books related to aspartame, click the link For More Info at aspartameexperiment.com.

Endnotes

The following subsections provide notes for each part of this report.

How this Report Came to Be

1. Name withheld, from e-mail to the author, 17 November 2005.
2. Russell L. Blaylock, MD, as quoted in the documentary *Sweet Remedy, the World Reacts to an Adulterated Food Supply* (Sound and Fury Productions, Inc., 2006).
3. Ajinomoto, filed by Shaun Weston, "Ajinomoto brands aspartame 'AminoSweet,'" FoodBev.com, 17 November 2009, http://www.foodbev.com/news/ajinomoto-brands-aspartame-aminosweet.
4. Russell L. Blaylock, MD, *Excitotoxins, the Taste that Kills* (Santa Fe, NM: Health Press, 1997).
5. Jerome Bressler, MD, *The Bressler Report*, http://www.sweetpoison.com/articles/fda-report-on-searle1.html; formally an *Establishment Inspection Report* (EIR) written by Dr. Bressler for the FDA, 1977.
6. Bressler, 1977.
7. See *FDA Audit - The Bressler Report*, at http://www.dorway.com/indexnew.htm#atwork.

Chapter 1: My Aspartame Experiment

1. Mark Gold, FDA Docket Submittal # 02P-0317, "Recall Aspartame as a Neurotoxic Drug: File #8: Aspartame & Human Studies." See http://www.fda.gov/ohrms/dockets/dailys/03/Jan03/012203/02P-0317_emc-000203.txt. References Ralph G. Walton in an interview by Mike Wallace broadcast on "60 Minutes," *CBS News*, 29 December 1996.
2. Bressler, 1977.
3. Ajinomoto, 2009.
4. See all industry sponsored studies listed at http://www.dorway.com/industry.html.
5. See all independent studies listed at http://www.dorway.com/nonindus.html.

Chapter 2: My Experimental Protocol

1. Joe Graedon and Teresa Graedon, PhD, *Deadly Drug Interactions, The People's Pharmacy Guide* (New York, NY: St. Martin's Griffin, 1995), 1.

2. Dr. Morando Soffritti, "Acesulfame Potassium: Soffritti Responds," *Environmental Health Perspectives*, July 2006. See http://www.pubmedcentral.nih.gov/articlerender.fcgi?artid=1570058.

3. Lewis D. Steginek and L.J. Filer, Jr., editors, *Aspartame, Physiology and Biochemistry* (New York, NY: Marcel Dekker, Inc.,1984), 292-294. Steginek and Filer are with the University of Iowa College of Medicine, Iowa City, Iowa.

4. Ibid., submitted by G. D. Searle & Co. to the FDA, Hearing Clerk File, Administrative Record, Aspartame 75F-0355, FDA, Rockville, MD.

5. Ibid., submitted by G. D. Searle & Co. to the FDA, Hearing Clerk File, Administrative Record, Aspartame 75F-0355, FDA, Rockville, MD. Also see File E-33, appendix to File E-34; File E-87 (1975), SC-18862: *A Supplemental Evaluation of Rat Brains from Two Tumorigenicity Studies*, PT 1227; and File E-70 (1974), SC-18862: *Lifetime Toxicity Study in the Rat*, PT 892H72, Final Report.

6. Ibid., submitted by G. D. Searle & Co. to the FDA, Hearing Clerk File, Administrative Record, Aspartame 75F-0355, FDA, Rockville, MD. Also see File E-36 (1973): *46-Week Oral Toxicity Study in the Hamster, Supplement; No. 1, Parts I and II.*

7. Ibid., submitted by G. D. Searle & Co. to the FDA, Hearing Clerk File, Administrative Record, Aspartame 75F-0355, FDA, Rockville, MD.

8. W.A. Reynolds, L.D. Steginek, L.J. Filer, Jr., and E. Renn, "Aspartame administration to the infant monkey: Hypothalamic morphology and plasma amino acid levels," *The Anatomical Record* 198: 73-85.

9. U.S. Senate proceedings, 1987, p 498.

10. See http://www.ramazzini.it/fondazione/docs/NYAS_Coca-Cola_Ramazzini.pdf.

11. Cori Bracket, *Sweet Misery: A Poisoned World: An industry case study of a food supply in crisis* (Sound and Fury Productions, 2001).

12. Ralph G. Walton, MD, "The Possible Role of Aspartame in Seizure Induction," in *Dietary Phenylalanine and Brain Function* (Boston, MA: Birkhauser, 1988), 159-168, compiled and edited by Richard Wurtman, MD.

13. Jeffrey A.Stamp and Theodore P. Labuza, "An Ion-Pair High Performance Liquid Chromatographic Method for the Determination of Aspartame and its Decomposition Products," *Journal of Food Science*, V 54, N 4 (1989): 1043-1046. Referenced by Mark D. Gold in a letter written on 4 December 1995 to Alan Paul, Editor-In-Chief, *Muscular Development Fitness Health* magazine, http://www.getbig.com/magazine/musdev/mdev9607.htm, regarding a review of Dr. Leibovitz' article on the safety of aspartame in the April 1995 issue of the magazine. Full contents of Gold's letter can be found at http://www.holistic-med.net/aspartame/aspartame.txt.

14. Steginek and Filer, 292-294.

15. Ibid., 407.

16. Dr. Christian Tschanz, Dr. Harriett H. Butchko, Dr. W. Wayne Stargel, and Dr. Frank N. Kotsonis, *The Clinical Evaluation of a Food Additive: Assessment of Aspartame* (New York, NY: CRC Press, 1996), 72.

17. Russell L. Blaylock, MD, *Excitotoxins, Neurodegeneration and Neurodevelopment*. See http://www.dorway.com/blayenn.html.

18. Data extracted and redrawn from Tschanz et al., 74.

19. Tschanz et al., 72.

20. Ibid.

21. Dr. Norm A. Sakow, DC, interview with author, May 2006.

22. Rowan Scarborough, *Rumsfeld's War: The Untold Story of America's Anti-Terrorist Commander* (Washington, DC: Regnery Publishing, Inc., 2004), 87.

23. Donna Voetee, *Supermarket Survival* (CD), V I, "Artificial Sweeteners," Part I, Aspartame; referring to *EXHIBIT 1, Objections of the National Soft Drink Association to a Final Rule Permitting the use of Aspartame in Carbonated Beverages and Carbonated Beverage Syrup Bases and a Request for a Hearing on the Objections*, Docket No. 82F-0305, 28 July 1983. The National Soft Drink Association has since changed its name to the American Beverage Association. See http://www.ameribev.org/index.aspx.

24. "Food Additives Permitted for Direct Addition to Food: Aspartame," *Federal Register*, 48 (8 July 1983): 31376-31382; Gold, 1995.

25. See www.militaryspot.com/gulf-war-syndrome.htm.

26. Morando Soffritti, Fiorella Belpoggi, Eva Tibaldi, Davide Degli Esposti, and Michelina Lauriola, "Life-Span Exposure to Low Doses of Aspartame Beginning during Prenatal Life Increases Cancer Effects in Rats," *Environmental Health Perspectives*, V115, N 9 (Sept

2007), http://www.ehponline.org/docs/2007/10271/abstract.html/, referencing the 2005 study done by the Cesare Maltoni Cancer Research Center, European Ramazzini Foundation of Oncology and Environmental Sciences.

27. Stegink and Filer, 406.

28. Center for the Evaluation of Risks to Human Reproduction, National Toxicology Program, U.S. Department of Health and Human Services, *NTP-CERHR Expert Panel Report on Reproductive and Developmental Toxicity of Methanol* (July 2001), 6. From the NIH website http://cerhr.niehs.nih.gov/chemicals/methanol/methanol_draft.pdf.

29. National Cancer Institute, U.S. National Institutes of Health, "Aspartame and Cancer: Questions and Answers," http://www.cancer.gov/cancertopics/factsheet/AspartameQandA, accessed 26 February 2007.

30. Soffritti et al., 2007.

31. Aspartame Information Center, http://www.aspartame.org/aspartame_facts_brochure.html, accessed 26 February 2007.

32. See http://notmilk.com/.

33. Aspartame Information Center, http://www.aspartame.org/, accessed 12 June 2007.

34. Soffritti et al., 2007.

35. Soffritti, "Acesulfame Potassium", 2006.

36. Dr. Morando Soffritti et al., "Mega-experiments to Identify and Assess Diffuse Carcinogenic Risks," *Annals of the New York Academy of Sciences*, 1999, http://www.annalsnyas.org/cgi/content/abstract/895/1/34?ck/=nck, accessed 21 July 2007.

37. Dr. Morando Soffritti et al., "European Ramazzini Foundation Stands Behind Aspartame Study Results, Announces Ongoing Research on Artificial Sweeteners," *La Leva di Archimede, Association for Freedom of Choice and Correct Information*, 5 May 2006, http://laleva.org/eng/2006/05/european_ramazzini_foundation_stands_behind_aspartame_study_results_announces_ongoing_research_on_artificial_sweeteners.html, accessed 21 July 2007.

38. Ibid.

39. Ibid.

40. "Scientists' New Study Affirms the Safety of Aspartame," *Nutrition Horizon, Health and Nutrition News*, 11 July 2007. See http://www.nutritionhorizon.com/newsmaker_article.asp?idNewsMaker=14458&fSite=AO545&next=6.

41. Tschanz et al., 61.

42. Ibid., 70.

43. Ibid., 108.

44. Ibid., 118.

45. Ibid., 131.

46. Ibid., 142.

47. Ibid., 155.

48. Ibid., 164.

49. Ibid., 175.

50. Jay Phelan and Terry Burnham, *Mean Genes* (Cambridge, MA: Perseus Publishing, 2000), 159.

51. Jay Phelan, from e-mail to the author, 10 September 2006.

52. Kaytee Products, Inc., Chilton, WI, www.kaytee.com.

Chapter 3: Resulting Tumors

1. "Everything You Need to Know About Aspartame," http://www.ific.org/publications/brochures/aspartamebroch.cfm, accessed 13 December 2007.

2. "About the International Food Information Council (IFIC) Foundation," http://www.ific.org/about/index.cfm, accessed 14 December 2007.

3. Morando Soffritti, Fiorella Belpoggi, Davide Degli Esposti, and Luca Lambertini, "L'aspartame induce linfomi e leucemie nei ratti" ("Aspartame induces lymphoma and leukemia in rats"), *European Journal of Oncology*, V 10, N 2 (2005). Study done at the Cesare Maltoni Cancer Research Center, European Ramazzini Foundation of Oncology and Environmental Sciences, Bologna, Italy.

4. Morando Soffritti, Fiorella Belpoggi, Eva Tibaldi, Davide Degli Esposti, and Michelina Lauriola, "Life-Span Exposure to Low Doses of Aspartame Beginning during Prenatal Life Increases Cancer Effects in Rats," *Environmental Health Perspectives,* V 115, N 9 (September 2007), http://www.ehponline.org/docs/2007/10271/abstract.html/, referencing the 2005 study done by the Cesare Maltoni Cancer Research Center, European Ramazzini Foundation of Oncology and Environmental Sciences.

5. B. A. Magnuson, G. A. Burdock, J. Doull, R. M. Kroes, G. M. Marsh, M. W. Pariza, P. S. Spencer, W. J. Waddell, R. Walker, and G. M. Williams, "Aspartame: A Safety Evaluation Based on Current Use Levels, Regulations, and Toxicological and Epidemiological Studies," *Critical Reviews in Toxicology,* September 2007, http://www.cspinet.org/new/pdf/aspartame912.pdf, accessed 30 July 2008.

6. Mark Gold, "Aspartame and Manufacturer-Funded Scientific Reviews," http://www.holisticmed.com/aspartame/burdock/, accessed 30 July 2008.

7. Unhee Lim, Amy F. Subar, Traci Mouw, Patricia Hartge, Lindsay M. Morton, Rachael Stolzenberg-Solomon, David Campbell, Albert R. Hollenbeck and Arthur Schatzkin, "Consumption of Aspartame-Containing Beverages and Incidence of Hematopoietic and Brain Malignancies," Division of Cancer Epidemiology and Genetics, Division of Cancer Control and Population Sciences, National Cancer Institute, NIH, Department of Health and Human Services, Information Management Services, Inc., Rockville, MD; and AARP, Washington, DC, *Cancer Epidemiology Biomarkers & Prevention,* V 15 (2006): 1654-1659. See http://cebp.aacrjournals.org/cgi/content/full/15/9/1654, accessed 4 August 2008.

8. Alan Kristal, Ulrike Peters, and John Potter, "Is It Time to Abandon the Food Frequency Questionnaire?" *Cancer Epidemiology Biomarkers & Prevention,* V 14 (December 2005): 2826-2828. See http://cebp.aacrjournals.org/cgi/content/full/14/12/2826, accessed 4 August 2008. Kristal et al. are with the Cancer Prevention Program, Fred Hutchinson Cancer Research Center, Seattle, Washington.

9. Unhee et al., 2006.

10. Ginger Cardinal, *The Rat: Guide to a Happy Healthy Pet* (Hoboken, NJ: Howell Book House, Wiley Publishing, Inc., 1998), 96.

Chapter 4: Other Adverse Results

1. Dr. Blaylock speaking in the documentary *Sweet Remedy,* 2006.
2. Ajinomoto, 2009.
3. H.J. Roberts, MD, *Aspartame Disease, an Ignored Epidemic* (West Palm Beach, FL: Sunshine Sentinel Press, Inc., 2001). See index listings under "Neurologic complications."
4. Name withheld, from e-mail to the author, 8 July 2006.
5. Blaylock, *Excitotoxins: The Taste That Kills,* xxi.
6. See http://www.emedicine.com/orthoped/byname/torticollis.htm.
7. See http://www.emedicine.com/emerg/topic597.htm#section~introduction.
8. Roberts, 1997: 250. In reference to K. Hyland, J.S. Fryburg, W.G. Wilson, et al., "Oral phenylalanine loading in dopa-responsive dystonia," *Neurology* 48 (1997): 1290-1297.
9. Lisa G. Jenkins and Betty Martini, "Mother Used Aspartame During Pregnancy," December 2000, http://www.rense.com/general6/motherused.htm.
10. David Austin, "Cerebral Palsy Symptoms - Clues to Identifying Cerebral Palsy," ezine articles, http://ezinearticles.com/?Cerebral-Palsy-Symptoms---Clues-to-Identifying-Cerebral-Palsy&id=1946113.
11. James Bowen, MD, and Arthur M. Evangelista, *Brain Cell Damage From Amino Acid Isolates: A Primary Concern From Aspartame-Based Products and Artificial Sweetening Agents,* May 2002, http://www.wnho.net/aspartame_brain_damage.htm. Evangelista is a former FDA investigator;
12. Betty Martini, from e-mail to the author, 30 May 2008.

13. Janet Starr Hull, *Sweet Poison: How the World's Most Popular Artificial Sweetener is Killing Us: My Story* (Far Hills, NJ: New Horizon Press, 1999), 269-270; referencing Louis J. Elsas, II, MD, Professor of Pediatrics, "Statement for the Labor and Human Resources Committee, U.S. Senate," *Congressional Record*, 3 November 1987.

14. Name withheld, from e-mail to the author, 11 May 2006.

15. Christine Lydon, MD, "Could There Be Evils Lurking in Aspartame Consumption?" http://www.aspartamekills.com/lydon.htm, reprinted from *Oxygen Magazine*, Robert Kennedy Publishing.

16. James Bowen, MD, "Aspartame in Chewing Gum," http://www.wnho.net/aspartame_chewing_gum.htm, posted 27 May 2005.

17. Name withheld, from e-mail to the author.

18. Janet Starr Hull, "Aspartame Side Effects," http://www.sweetpoison.com/aspartame-side-effects.html. Hull is creator of the Aspartame Detox Program.

19. Roberts, 2001: 463, 467, 822, and 823.

20. Ibid., 466. References J.R. Norris, G.G. Meadows, L.K. Massey, et al., "Tyrosine- and phenylalanine-restricted formula diet augments immunocompetence in healthy humans," *American Journal of Clinical Nutrition* 51 (1990): 188-196.

21. Ibid., 466. References R.W. Wannemacher, A.S. Klainer, R.E. Dinterman, and W.R. Beisel, "The significance and mechanism of an increased serum phenylalanine-tyrosine ratio during infection," *American Journal of Clinical Nutrition* 29 (1967): 997-1006.

22. L.J. Filer, Jr., and Lewis D. Stegink, "Effect of Aspartame on Plasma Phenylalanine Concentration in Humans," in *Dietary Phenylalanine and Brain Function*, edited by R.J. Wurtman and E. Ritter-Walker, Washington DC (May 1987): 19.

23. M.S. Schuett, RD, *National PKU News*, "Questions and Answers about PKU," Fall 1997, http://www.pkunews.org/about/question.htm.

24. Hugh A. Tilson, Dayao Zhao, N. John Peterson, Kevin Nanry, and J.-S. Hong, "Behavioral and Neurological Effects of Aspartame," in *Dietary Phenylalanine and Brain Function*, edited by R.J. Wurtman and E. Ritter-Walker, Washington DC (May 1987): 104-105.

25. Matthew J. During, Ian N. Acworth, and Richard J. Wurtman, "An In Vivo Study of Dopamine Release in Striatum: The Effects of Phenylalanine," in *Proceedings of the First International Meeting on Dietary Phenylalanine and Brain Function*, edited by R.J. Wurtman and E. Ritter-Walker, Washington DC (May 1987): 81.

26. "Foods high in tyrosine, http://www.nutritional-supplements-health-guide.com/tyrosine-foods.html

27. Blaylock, 1997: 18

28. Ibid: 25

29. J.M. Bjork, D.M. Dougherty, F.G. Moeller, "A positive correlation between self-ratings of depression and laboratory-measured aggression," Department of Psychiatry and Behavioral Sciences, University of Texas, Houston, Texas, USA, http://cat.inist.fr/?aModele=afficheN&cpsidt=2788501.

30. A. Srikumar Menon, Ann L. Gruber-Baldini, J. Richard Hebel, Bruce Kaup, David Loreck, Sheryl Itkin Zimmerman, Lynda Burton, Pearl German, Jay Magaziner, "Relationship between aggressive behaviors and depression among nursing home residents with dementia," Mental Health Clinical Center, Veterans Affairs Maryland Health Care Center, MD, USA, http://www3.interscience.wiley.com/journal/77002070/abstract?CRETRY=1&SRETRY=0.

31. Erling Roland, "Aggression, depression, and bullying others," Centre for Behavioural Research, Stavanger University College, Stavanger, Norway, http://www3.interscience.wiley.com/journal/92013843/abstract?CRETRY=1&SRETRY=0

32. Kelly Brown, Geraldine Shaw, "Juvenile Depression and Aggression: Is There a Linkage," paper presented at a Meeting of the Kentucky Psychological Association, 8 November 1997, http://eric.ed.gov/ERICWebPortal/custom/portlets/recordDetails/detailmini.jsp?_nfpb=true&_&ERICExtSearch_SearchValue_0=ED420403&ERICExt Search_SearchType_0=no&accno=ED420403.

33. See http://www.rxlist.com/cgi/generic/stalevo_cp.htm.

34. Blaylock, 1997: "About the Author," last page of book.

35. Ibid: 18.

36. Andrea Byrd, "Serotonin and Its Uses," http://serendip.brynmawr.edu/bb/neuro/neuro99/web1/Byrd.html.

37. Blaylock, 1997: 25-26.

38. C Nemeroff, "Effects of Tryptophan Depletion on Aggression in Men," *Neuropsychopharmacology*, April 2000; online at Psychiatry Journal Watch, 22 August 2000, http://psychiatry.jwatch.org/cgi/content/citation/2000/822/2.

39. J.M. Bjork, Donald M. Dougherty, F.Gerald Moeller, Alan C. Swann, Department of Psychiatry and Behavioral Sciences University of Texas-Houston Medical School, Houston, TX, "Differential behavioral effects of plasma tryptophan depletion and loading in aggressive and nonaggressive men," *Neuropsychopharmacology,* V 22, N 4: 357-369. Published online by Nature Publishing, New York, NY, 1987, http://cat.inist.fr/?aModele=afficheN&cpsidt=1315612.

40. J.M. Bjork, Donald M. Dougherty, F.Gerald Moeller, Don R. Cherek, Alan C. Swann, Department of Psychiatry and Behavioral Sciences University of Texas-Houston Medical School, Houston, TX, "The effects of tryptophan depletion and loading on laboratory aggression in men: time course and a food-restricted control," *Neuropsychopharmacology,* February 1999, V 142, N 1: 24-30. Online at http://www.springerlink.com/content/1av3kh7kb2lkh5bl/.

41. Dawn M. Marsh, Donald M. Dougherty, F. Gerard Moeller, Alan C. Swann, Ralph Spiga, Department of Psychiatry & Behavioral Sciences, University of Texas Health Science Center at Houston, Houston, TX, "Laboratory-Measured Aggressive Behavior of Women: Acute Tryptophan Depletion and Augmentation," Neuropsychopharmacology (2002) V.26: 660-671. Online at http://www.ncbi.nlm.nih.gov/pubmed/11927191.

42. Ibid

43. Cori Bracket, 2001.

44. See "Graves Disease" under the "Hypothyroidism" bullet, at http://www.emedicine-health.com/thyroid_problems/page2_em.htm.

45. Charles Miller, posted message regarding Dr. Janet Starr Hull, "FW: Dr. Hull and Graves Disease," 14 June 2004, http://www.bio.net/bionet/mm/toxicol/2004-June/--3495.html.

46. See http://myaspartameexperiment.com/index.php? page = 4.

47. Name withheld, from e-mail to the author, 1 January 2005.

48. U.S. Senate proceedings, 1987.

49. Stoddard, Mary, "Before You Reach for That Sweetener!" 6 November 1996, misc.healthdiabetes newsgroup. Stoddard is founder of the Aspartame Consumer Safety Network (ACSN).

50. Carol Guilford, from e-mail to the author, 23 June 2006.

51. See http://www.presidiotex.com/92symptoms/ and http://www.presidiotex.com/aspartame/Facts/92_Symptoms/92_symptoms.html.

52. Courtnee M., South Dakota, http://presidiotex.com/personal_stories/Diet_Croak_Addict/diet_croak_addict.html.

53. "nutrasweet? 2 June 2006, Hair loss resulting from the use of NutraSweet, http://www.keratin.net/forums/viewtopic.php?p=42456.

54. Cardinal, 1998.

55. World Health Organization, "Toxicological Evaluation of Some Enzymes, Modified Starches and Certain Other Substances," *WHO Food Additives Series, N 1*, 1972, http://www.inchem.org/documents/jecfa/jecmono/v001je21.htm.

56. C. Trocho, R. Pardo, I. Rafecas, J. Virgili, X. Remesar, J.A. Fernandez-Lupez, and M. Alemany, "Formaldehyde derived from dietary aspartame binds to tissue components in vivo," Department de Bioquimica i Biologia Molecular, Facultat de Biologia, Universitat de Barcelona, Spain, PubMed, 1998, http://www.ncbi.nlm.nih.gov/pubmed/9714421, accessed 5 August 2008.

57. "Formaldehyde Accumulation Seen from Ingested Aspartame," http://www.ethical-investing.com/monsanto/news/10002.htm, accessed 25 August 2008.

58. Rich Murray, "Formaldehyde as a potent unexamined cofactor in cancer research—sources include methanol, dark wines and liquors, aspartame, wood and tobacco smoke," May 2007, http://www.nabble.com/formaldehyde-as-a-potent-unexamined-cofactor-in-cancer-research----sources-include-methanol,-dark-wines-and-liquors,-aspartame,-wood-and-tobacco-smoke:-IARC-Monographs-on-the-Evaluation-of-Carcinogenic-Risks-to-Humans-implicate-formaldehyde-in--88-and-alc-td10323241.html.

59. Indya Gordon, e-mail forwarded to the FDA, "Subject: FW: Tordoff: aspartame doesn't increase hunger & weight 6.9.99," http://www.fda.gov/ohrms/DOCKETS/dailys/03/May03/050803/94f-0405-emc0259.txt.

Chapter 5: Conclusion

1. Tschanz et al., Preface.
2. Ibid., 26.
3. Ajinomoto, 2009.
4. Kerry Mahoney, DVM, *Pathology Report*, County of San Diego, Department of Agriculture Weights and Measures, Animal Disease Diagnostic Laboratory, San Diego, California, 29 March 2007.
5. Alexandra Silber, DVM, *Pathology Report*, County of San Diego, Department of Agriculture Weights and Measures, Animal Disease Diagnostic Laboratory, San Diego, California, 14 May 2007.
6. Silber, *Pathology Report*, 11 June 2007.
7. Roberts, 2001, 673.
8. U.S. Environmental Protection Agency (EPA), "Formaldehyde, CASRN 50-00-0," http://www.epa.gov/iris/subst/0419.htm.
9. Sharon G. Adler, Jan J. Weening, "A Case of Acute Renal Failure," Harbor-UCLA Medical Center, Division of Nephrology and Hypertension, Torrance, California; Academic Medical Center, Amsterdam, Netherlands, *Clinical Journal of the American Society of Nephrology 1: 158-165*, 2006; http://cjasn.asnjournals.org/cgi/content/full/1/1/158.
10. Roberts, 2001, 673.
11. "The Truth about Aspartame," http://www.aspartametruth.net/.
12. Tschanz et al., 24.
13. Midge Decter, "Rumsfeld: A Personal Portrait," Harper Collins Publishers Inc., NY, NY; 2003: 80-89.
14. Farber, Steven A., "Aspartame and the Regulation of Food Additives: A Study of FDA Decision-Making and a Proposal for Change," Thesis for Master of Science in Technology and Public Policy at Massachusetts Institute of Technology, Cambridge, MA 02139; 1989: 38.
15. Roberts, 2001: 88. In reference to L. Tollefson, R.J. Barnard, and W.H. Glinsmann, "Monitoring of adverse reactions to aspartame reported to the U.S. Food and Drug Administration," in *Proceedings of the First International Meeting on Dietary Phenylalanine and Brain Function*, edited by R.J. Wurtman and E. Ritter-Walker, Washington DC (May 1987): 347-372.
16. Aspartame Information Center, http://www.aspartame.org/, accessed 12 June 2007.

Appendix A: What is Aspartame?

1. Aspartame Information Center, http://www.aspartame.org/aspartame_faq.html, accessed 12 June 2007.
2. Betty Martini, from e-mail to the author, 1 July 2006.
3. Ajinomoto, 2009.
4. Aspartame Information Center, http://www.aspartame.org/.
5. Blend of sugar, aspartame-based Equal, and acesulfame potassium. See http://pqasb.pqarchiver.com/newsday/access/764391081.html?dids=764391081:764391081&FMT=ABS&FMTS=ABS:FT&date=Dec+15%2C+2004&author=&pub=Newsday&edition=Combined+editions&startpage=B.68&desc=HOLIDAY+BAKING%2C+The+skinny+on+low-calorie+sugar+blends.

6. Equal, Equal Measure, Canderel (blend of aspartame and acesulfame-K), Sweetex and Peptis are marketed by Merisant UK Ltd. Mivida is sold in Italy. Equal is sold in the USA, Eastern Europe, South Africa and India. Sweetex and Peptis are sold in Poland. See http://www.canderel.uk.com/scripts/FR1.HTM.

7. Natrasweet is marketed in Brazil.

8. See http://www.natrataste.com.

9. Kroger Sweet Servings is manufactured by the Kroger Company, Cincinnati, OH.

10. Sugar Twin Plus is a blend of aspartame and saccharin marketed by Alberto Culver, Melrose Park, IL.

11. Twinsweet - Sweet Inspiration is an aspartame-acesulfame salt from the Holland Sweetener Company, the largest European manufacturer of aspartame.

12. Miwon is manufactured by Miwon USA, Inc., and Miwon Trading & Shipping Co., Ltd., South Korea. See http://my.ecplaza.net/miwontrading/1.asp.

13. NutraSweet, NutraSweet Spoonfuls and Neotame (an enhanced derivative of aspartame 8,000 times sweeter than sugar, approved by FDA in 2002) are marketed by the NutraSweet Company, previously a subsidiary of Monsanto. Investment firm J.W. Childs bought NutraSweet from Monsanto in 2000. See http://biz.yahoo.com/ic/101/101064.html.

14. Sanecta and Tri-Sweet are listed as alternative trade names for aspartame at http://ntp-server.niehs.nih.gov/index.cfm?objectid=03E4FDB1-CCE9-970E-0455D3DC53465EA7.

15. In the European Union, aspartame is known under its additive code, E951. See http://encyclopedia.thefreedictionary.com/E951.

16. NouriSweet, marketed by Fenchem in Europe, contains Aspartame, Acesulfame-K & Erythritol. See http://www.foodnavigator.com/news-by-product/productpresentation.asp?id=553&k=nourisweet-trade-branded.

17. Aspartame brand sweetener is marketed by Albertsons.

18. Ajinomoto, 2009.

19. See http://www.greenfacts.org/aspartame/l-3/aspartame-1.htm.

20. See http://encyclopedia.thefreedictionary.com/E951.

21. See http://www.chemindustry.com/chemicals/78480.html.

22. Aspartame is considered chemically synonymous with the following chemical compounds: 1-Methyl N-L-alpha-aspartyl-L-phenylalanate; 1-Methyl N-L-alpha-aspartyl-L-phenylalanine; 22839-47-0; 3-Amino-4-[(1-benzyl-2-methoxy-2-oxoethyl) amino]-4-oxobutanoic acid; 3-Amino-N-(alpha-carboxyphenethyl) succinamic acid N-methyl ester; 3-Amino-N-(alpha-carboxyphenethyl) succinamic acid N-methyl ester, stereoisomer; 3-Amino-N-(alpha-methoxycarbonylphenethyl) succinamic acid; 53906-69-7; 7421-84-3; APM; Asp-phe-ome; Aspartam [INN-French]; Aspartame, L,L-alpha-; Aspartamo [INN-Spanish]; Aspartamum [INN-Latin]; Aspartyl-phenylalanine methyl ester; C11045; CCRIS 5456; CHEMBANK832325; Dipeptide sweetener; EINECS 245-261-3; HSDB 3915; L-Aspartyl-L-phenylalanine methyl ester; L-Phenylalanine, L-alpha-aspartyl-, 2-methyl ester; L-Phenylalanine, N-L-alpha-aspartyl-, 1-methyl ester; Methyl aspartylphenylalanate; Methyl L-alpha-aspartyl-L-phenylalanate; Methyl L-aspartyl-L-phenylalanine; Methyl N-L-alpha-aspartyl-L-phenylalaninate; N-L-alpha-Aspartyl-L-phenylalanine 1-methyl ester; N-L-alpha-Aspartyl-L-phenylalanine methyl ester; SC 18862; SC-18862; Succinamic acid, 3-amino-N-(alpha-carboxyphenethyl)- N-methyl ester, stereoisomer; and Sweet dipeptide. See http://www.chemindustry.com/chemicals/78480.html.

23. See http://encyclopedia.thefreedictionary.com/E951.

24. See http://www.greenfacts.org/aspartame/l-3/aspartame-1.htm.

25. See http://www.ncchem.com/snftaas/aldehydes.htm#ASPARTAME.

Appendix B: Does Aspartame Make You Fat?

1. Barbara Kantrowitz and Pat Wingert, "Why Women Lose Weight—or Don't," *Newsweek*, 4 December 2007, http://www.newsweek.com/id/73765?GT1=10645.

2. Stegink and Filer, iv. Refers to *Federal Register* 46 (1981): 38285, and *Federal Register* 48 (1983): 21378.

3. Mark Gold and Rich Murray, "Merisant aspartame sales plummet in 2005," 4 April 2006, http://rmforall.blogspot.com/2006/04/merisant-aspartame-sales-plummet-in.html. Refers to Merisant's annual report at sec.gov/Archives/edgar/data/1270597/000110465906020777/a06-7464_110k.htm.

4. "Obesity epidemic in U.S. kids may have peaked: Study offers 'first encouraging finding' after a 25-year-increase in weight," *The Associated Press*, 27 May 2008, http://www.msnbc.msn.com/id/24842630.

5. Daniel DeNoon, MD, "Drink More Diet Soda, Gain More Weight—Overweight Risk Soars 41% With Each Daily Can of Diet Soft Drink," WebMD Medical News, 13 June 2005, http://my.webmd.com/content/Article/107/108476.htm.

6. Dr. Russell Blaylock, "Obesity Secret Ignored," November 2007, http://www.rense.com/general79/obesity.htm.

7. Liancheng Zhao et al., Fu Wai Hospital and Cardiovascular Institute, Chinese Academy of Medical Sciences, Beijing China, and researchers from Northwestern University in Chicago, and the INTERMAP Cooperative Research Group, "UNC Researchers Find MSG Use Linked To Obesity," http://www.eurekalert.org/pub_releases/2008-08/uonc-urf081308.php#, accessed 25 August 2008.

8. Blaylock, 2007.

9. Ibid

10. Ibid

11. Ibid

12. Ibid

13. Jack L. Samuels, "The Obesity Epidemic: Should We Believe What We Read and Hear," originally printed in *Wise Traditions*, V 5, N 2 (Summer 2004), http://www.truthinlabeling.org/obesityepidemic.html.

14. Blaylock, 2007.

15. Ibid

16. Ibid

17. Ibid

18. Ibid

19. Ibid

20. See www.thegardendiet.com/news/demi.html.

Appendix C: Is Aspartame Addictive?

1. H. J. Roberts, M.D., F.A.C.P., F.C.C.P., "Aspartame (NutraSweet) Addiction," *Townsend Letter for Doctors*; V 198 (January 2000): 52-57, http://www.dorway.com/tldaddic.html.

2. Ibid

3. Peter C., "Alcohol, addiction, rehabilitation, detoxification," http://stanford.wellsphere.com/complementary-alternative-medicine-article/alcohol-addiction-rehabilitation-detoxification/453354.

4. Jackson, "Is Diet Cola Bad for Alcoholics, Addicts?," http://cleanandsoberissexy.com/is-diet-cola-bad-for-alcoholics-addicts/.

5. Roberts 2000.

6. ibid

7. "Methanol," http://www.nationmaster.com/encyclopedia/alcoholic-beverage.

8. "Alcohol facts," Addiction, Science, Research, and Education Center, University of Texas, Austin, http://www.utexas.edu/research/asrec/alcoholfacts.html.

9. Akram Askar, Abdulkarim Al-Suwaida, "Methanol Intoxication with Brain Hemorrhage: Catastrophic outcome of late presentation," Division of Nephrology, Department of Medicine, King Khalid University Hospital, Riyadh, Saudi Arabia; *Saudi Journal of Kidney Diseases and Transplantation*, 2007, V 18: 117-22, http://www.sjkdt.org/article.asp?issn=1319-2442;year=2007;volume=18;issue=1;spage=117;epage=122;aulast=Askar.

10. Bio-Medicine, http://www.bio-medicine.org/q-more/medicine-dictionary/alcohol/.

11. Askar et.al, 2007.

12. Ibid

13. B. Amarnath, "Addiction to Alcohol," http://en.allexperts.com/q/Addiction-Alcohol-2053/Alcohol-Poisoning.htm.

14. "Methanol Poisoning Overview," http://www.antizol.com/mpoisono.htm.

15. Askar et.al, 2007

16. Forum: "A Second Look at Methanol," *Environmental Health Perspectives*, V 101, N 2, June 1993, http://www.ehponline.org/docs/1993/101-2/forum.html.

17. Ibid

18. Roberts 2000.

19. Dr. Woodrow C. Monte, "Aspartame: Methanol and the Public Health," *Journal of Applied Nutrition*, V 36, N 1, 1984, p 1. See http://www.sweetpoison.com/articles/dr-woodrow-monte.html.

20. Methanol, Wikipedia, http://en.wikipedia.org/wiki/Methanol

21. ©Ajinomoto Food Ingredients LLC, http://www.aspartame.net/info/faq_is_methanol_a_problem.asp

22. Dr. James Duke, USDA, "Phytochemical and Ethnobotanical Databases," http://www.ars-grin.gov/duke/

23. Ibid, http://www.ars-grin.gov/cgi-bin/duke/farmacy2.pl?282

24. Monte, 1984, p 62; in reference to L.J. Zatmann; "The Effect of Ethanol on the Metabolism of Methanol in Man." *Biochemical Journal*, V 40: 67-68; 1946. See http://www.sweetpoison.com/articles/dr-woodrow-monte10.html.

25. Ibid: 2, 46; in reference to G.R. Bartlett; "Inhibition of Methanol Oxidation by Ethanol in the Rat." *American Journal of Physiology*, 1950; V 163: 619-621.

26. Alex Constantine, "NutraFear & NutraLoathing in Augusta, Georgia," *You Are Being Lied To: The Disinformation Guide to Media Distortion, Historical Whitewashes, and Cultural Myths* (an anthology edited by Russ Kick), The Disinformation Company Ltd., 2001, p 309.

27. "Embalming Techniques," http://www.embalming.net/.

28. "nucleus accumbens," Wikipedia, http://en.wikipedia.org/wiki/Nucleus_accumbens.

29. Ibid

30. R. Exley, M.A. Clements, H Hartung, J.M. McIntosh, S.J. Cragg, "Alpha6-containing nicotinic acetylcholine receptors dominate the nicotine control of dopamine neurotransmission in nucleus accumbens," Department of Physiology, Anatomy and Genetics, University of Oxford, Oxford, UK, http://www.ncbi.nlm.nih.gov/pubmed/18033235.

31. Christian A. Heidbreder, Michela Andreoli, Clara Marcon, Panayotis K. Thanos, Charles R. Ashby, Jr. and Eliot L. Gardner, "Role of dopamine D3 receptors in the addictive properties of ethanol," Center of Excellence for Drug Discovery in Psychiatry, GlaxoSmithKline Pharmaceuticals, Verona, Italy; Medical Department, Brookhaven National Laboratory, Upton, New York, USA; Department of Pharmaceutical Sciences, College of Pharmacy and Allied Health Professions, Saint John's University, Jamaica, New York, USA; Intramural Research Program, National Institute on Drug Abuse, Baltimore, Maryland, USA, *Drugs of Today*, 2004, V. 40 (4): 355-365, http://www.bnl.gov/thanoslab/Thanos%20PDF/Heidbreder_Drugs_Todaypdf.pdf.

32. Ibid

33. Ibid

34. Ibid

35. Dean D. Krahn, MD, "The Doctor will See You Now; Behavior: Rewards and Addictions," online October, 1999, http://www.thedoctorwillseeyounow.com/articles/behavior/rewards_1/.

36. Ibid

37. Ibid

Appendix D: Misinformation About My Experiment

1. Thomas Pynchon, *Gravity's Rainbow*, Viking Press, 1973, p 251, see http://en.wiki-quote.org/wiki/Thomas_Pynchon.

Appendix E: What They Say About My Experiment

1. Poster unknown; from http://purrl.net/view/comments/20123/my-aspartame-experi-mentcom/:
2. E-mail from Marjo Sukeva; Pori, Finland; 4/3/2008
3. E-mail from edward@naturalhealthstrategies.com
4. Scaredhuman; http://portland.indymedia.org/en/2008/02/372604.shtml; 2/21/2008
5. E-mail from Carol Guilford forwarding a post by Rich at http://www.rich-gautier.com; February 2008
6. E-mail from LalChumi Ralte; 3/11/2008
7. E-mail from Diane Kaste, Wheaton, IL; 2/20/2008
8. canUdi9it; "Woman Conducts Own Aspertame Study with Pet Rats;" http://digg.com/general_sciences/Woman_Conducts_Own_Aspertame_Study_With_Pet_Rats_PICS; 02/15/2008
9. cubicledropout; Ibid
10. scooterbaga; Ibid
11. r00k1200; Ibid
12. dimplemonkey; Ibid
13. lik3n; Ibid
14. JohnBoyer; Ibid
15. kyle90; Ibid
16. chemicalwahoo; Ibid
17. snugglebear; Ibid
18. Fratz; Ibid
19. nonsequitor; Ibid
20. Fratz; Ibid

Appendix F: Did I Fake My Data?

1. Michael Crichton, "Aliens Cause Global Warming," speech at California Institute of Technology, Pasadena, California, January 17, 2003, http://www.quoteland.com/author.asp?AUTHOR_ID=2132.
2. Roberts, 2001: 88.
3. Cardinal, *The Rat*, 97.
4. Jo Hartley, "NutraSweet - A Look at the History of Deception Behind Its Marketing (Part 2)," *Natural News*, http://www.naturalnews.com/023175.html, 6 May 2008.
5. "Animal Lifespans," http://www.pubquizhelp.com/animals/lifespan.html.
6. "Hidden Sources of Processed Free Glutamic Acid (MSG): Ingredients that Serve as Common MSG-Reaction Triggers," http://truthinlabeling.org/Jack_hiddensources.htm.
7. Hans-Peter Eck, Thomas Mertens, Heinrich Rosokat, Gerd Fätkenheuer, Christoph Pohl, Matthias Schrappe, Volker Daniel, Helmut Näher, Detlef Petzoldt, Peter Drings, Wulf Dröge "T4+ cell numbers are correlated with plasma glutamate and cystine levels: association of hyperglutamataemia with immunodeficiency in dis-eases with different aetiologies," *International Immunology*, V 4, N 1: 7-13, January 1992, http://intimm.oxfordjournals.org/cgi/content/abstract/4/1/7.
8. Dr. Betty Martini, "Winning the Aspartame War," September 2009, http://www.thenhf.com/articles/articles_977/articles_977.htm.
9. Hans-Peter Eck, et. al., 1992
10. "Cysteine and Cystine Functions," http://www.vitaminsdiary.com/amino-acids/cys-teine-cystine.htm.
11. Eck, et. al., 1992
12. "Dr. Duke's Phytochemical and Ethnobotanical Databases: Chemicals in: Camellia sinensis (L.) KUNTZE (Theaceae)—Tea," http://www.ars-grin.gov/cgi-bin/duke/farmacy2.pl?198.
13. David Tolson, "Theanine Science," http://www.goendurance.com/a96_Theanine_Science.html.

14. "Glutamate receptor," Wikipedia, http://en.wikipedia.org/wiki/Glutamate_receptor.

15. David Tolson, "Green Tea," http://www.goendurance.com/?ingredients_id=17.

16. "Micronutrient Information Center: Tea," Linus Pauling Institute, University of Oregon, http://lpi.oregonstate.edu/infocenter/phytochemicals/tea/.

17. Dr. David Duke, Ethnobotanical and Phytochemical Database, U.S.D.A., http://www.ars-grin.gov/duke/, (search for "chemicals and activities in a particular plant," select "tea" for the search).

18. Mary Shomon, "Green Tea Extract Increases Metabolism, May Aid in Weight Loss," 3 December 2003, http://thyroid.about.com/cs/dietweightloss/a/greentea.htm.

19. Shelley R. Kramer, "Common pesticides use fluoridation chemicals as their main ingredient," http://www.healthy-communications.com/fluoride-pesticides.htm.

20. Yi Lu, Wen-Fei Guo, Xian-Qiang Yang, Department of Tea Science and Department of Chemistry, Zhejiang University, People's Republic of China, "Fluoride Content in Tea and Its Relationship with Tea Quality," Journal of Agriculture and Food Chemistry, 2004, V 52, N 14: 4472–4476, http://pubs.acs.org/doi/abs/10.1021/jf0308354.

21. "Health effects of tea: Effects of fluoride," Wikipedia, http://en.wikipedia.org/wiki/Health_effects_of_tea.

22. Yi Lu, et. al; 2004.

23. "Health effects of tea: Effects of fluoride," Wikipedia, http://en.wikipedia.org/wiki/Health_effects_of_tea.

24. E. Malinowskaa, I. Inkielewiczb, W. Czarnowskib, P. Szefer, "Assessment of fluoride concentration and daily intake by human from tea and herbal infusions," *Food and Chemical Toxicology*, V 46, No 3, March 2008, 1055-1061, http://www.sciencedirect.com/science?_ob=ArticleURL&_udi=B6T6P-4R2H932-3&_user=10&_rdoc=1&_fmt=&_orig=search&_sort=d&_docanchor=&view=c&_acct=C000050221&_version=1&_urlVersion=0&_userid=10&md5=ad132aa5e9e64b226f34e4da98afa404.

25. Chris Recchia, Manager of Quality and Innovation, Salada Tea, "Salada: FAQ," http://www.greentea.com/faq.aspx.

26. Jia Hepeng, "China maps massive problem of water contamination," 29 April 2005, http://www.scidev.net/en/news/china-maps-massive-problem-of-water-contamination.html.

27. M. Dinesh Kumar, Tushaar Shah, "Groundwater Pollution and Contamination in India: The Emerging Challenge," International Water Management Institute, Nagar, India, http://www.iwmi.cgiar.org/iwmi-tata/files/pdf/ground-pollute4_FULL_.pdf.

28. "Tea," Wikipedia, http://en.wikipedia.org/wiki/Tea.

29. "Fluoride in Green Tea: Danger in Lipton Instant Iced Tea," http://www.amazing-green-tea.com/fluoride-in-green-tea.html.

30. E. Malinowskaa, et. al., 2008

31. Yi Lu, et. al; 2004.

32. "Traditional Medicinals, FAQS, Ingredients: Are your green teas tested for fluoride content?" Traditional Medicinals, http://www.traditionalmedicinals.com/FAQs_ingredients.

33. H.P. Carr, E. Lombi, H. Küpper, S.P. McGrath and M.H. Wong, "Accumulation and distribution of aluminium and other elements in tea (Camellia sinensis) leaves," *Agronomie.* V 23 (2003): 705-710, http://www.agronomy-journal.org/index.php?option=article&access=standard&Itemid=129&url=/articles/agro/abs/2003/07/A3717/A3717.html.

34. Dr. Russell Blaylock MD, "Why Fluoride is Toxic: The Toxic Effect of Fluoride and Aluminum," *The Blaylock Wellness Report: Living a Long, Healthy Life*, V 1, No 4, September 2004.

35. Dr. Russell Blaylock MD, "Miracle Tea Protects Your Heart and Brain While Preventing Cancer," *The Blaylock Wellness Report: Living a Long, Healthy Life*, V 4, No 8, August 2007.

36. "Hidden Sources of Processed Free Glutamic Acid (MSG): Addendum," http://truthinlabeling.org/Jack_addendum_R.html.

37. http://www.drugs.com/sfx/dextrose-side-effects.html.

38. "Sugar: Sweet by Nature," http://www.sugar.org/consumers/sweet_by_nature.asp?id=277.

39. Bart Kosko, Noise, Viking Press: Penguin Group, USA, 2006: 54-57.

40. Karen Lau, W. Graham McLean, Dominic P. Williams, C. Vyvyan Howard, "Synergistic interactions between commonly used food additives in a developmental neurotoxicity test," Toxicological Sciences, V 90, N 1, March 2006, http://toxsci.oxfordjournals.org/cgi/content/abstract/90/1/178.

41. J. Dich, S.H. Zahm, A. Hanberg, and H.O. Adami, Department of Cancer Epidemiology, Karolinska Institute and Radiumhemmet, Karolinska University Hospital, Stockholm Sweden. Published on PubMed at: http://www.ncbi.nlm.nih.gov/entrez/query.fcgi?cmd=Retrieve&db=pubmet&dopt=Abstract&List)uids=9498903.

42. Şükran Çakira and Rabia Sarikayab, "Genotoxicity testing of some organophosphate insecticides in the Drosophila wing spot test," Department of Biology, Kırıkkale University, Yahşihan, Kırıkkale, Turkey, and Department of Biology Education, Gazi University, Ankara, Turkey, Elsevier Ltd, 2004, http://www.sciencedirect.com/science?_ob=ArticleURL&_udi=B6T6P-4F60N87-1&_user=10&_rdoc=1&_fmt=&_orig=search&_sort=d&view=c&_acct=C000050221&_version=1&_urlVersion=0&_userid=10&md5=25c79c0727a1b08d76d35cfb726de1d1.

43. Mosby's Medical Dictionary, 8th edition, Elsevier, 2009, http://medical-dictionary.thefreedictionary.com/genotoxic.

44. The American Heritage® Science Dictionary, Houghton Mifflin Company, 2005, http://www.thefreedictionary.com/RNA.

45. "Pesticide use in the United States," Wikipedia, http://en.wikipedia.org/wiki/Pesticide_use_in_the_United_States.

46. "New Model Suggests Role of Low Vitamin D in Cancer Development," UC San Diego Medical Center Press Release. May 22, 2009, http://health.ucsd.edu/news/2009/5-22-vitamin-D-dinomit.htm.

47. Amy Coombs, "Corn Herbicide Atrazine Damages Human & Animal Immune System: New Curse for an Old Foe." Science Now Daily News, 8 December 06.

48. Shane Ellison - The People's Chemist, "Toxin in Corn," 25 August, 2008, http://thepeopleschemist.com/blog/index.php?s=toxin+in+corn.

49. Ibid

50. Coombs, 2006.

51. Dich, et. al.

52. Gregory M. Lamb, "When genetically modified plants go wild," Christian Science Monitor, 31 August 2006, http://www.csmonitor.com/2006/0831/p15s01-sten.html.

53. "Synthesis of L-aspartic acid by Escherichia coli and Pseudomonas fluorenscens as related to the cultivation conditions;" http://www.ncbi.nlm.nih.gov/entrez/query.fcgi?cmd=Retrieve&db=PubMed&list_uids=117446&dopt=Abstract; republished from Russian medical journal, Prikl Biokhim Mikrobiol, Sep-Oct 1979, V 15 N 5: 671-675.

54. Malofeeva IV, Iakovieva VI, "L-aspartic acid synthesis from ammonium fumarate by free and immobilized Escherichia coli cells;" http://www.ncbi.nlm.nih.gov/entrez/query.fcgi?itool=abstractplus&db=pubmed&cmd=Retrieve&dopt=abstractplus&list_uids=37496; originally published in Prikl Biokhim Mikrobiol, 1979; PMID: 37496.

55. "Kinetics mechanism of L-aspartate synthesis from ammonium fumarate catalyzed by free and immobilized cells of E. coli;" http://www.ncbi.nlm.nih.gov/entrez/query.fcgi?itool=abstractplus&db=pubmed&cmd=Retrieve&dopt=abstractplus&list_uids=7018589; originally published in Biokhimiia, 1980; PMID: 7018589.

56. United States Patent 5008190, http://www.freepatentsonline.com/5008190.html.

57. "Faecal bacteria," Lenntech Water Treatment Solutions, http://www.lenntech.com/faecal-bacteria.htm.

58. Malofeeva IV, et al., 1979

59. "Ion: Formation of polyatomic and molecular ions," Wikipedia, the free encyclopedia, http://en.wikipedia.org/wiki/Ion.

60. "Ammonia: Sources and Emissions," http://www.scorecard.org/chemical-profiles/html/ammonia.html.

61. Posted by Tiffany O'Callaghan, "E. Coli in the fountain soda supply?" *Time.com*, http://wellness.blogs.time.com/2010/01/12/e-coli-in-the-fountain-soda-supply/.

62. From an e-mail message received from Betty Martini on 30 April 2009.

63. Eyyüp Rencuzogullari, Berrin Ayaz Tuylu, Mehmet Topaktas, Hasan Basri Ila, Ahmet Kayraldiz, Mehmet Arslan, Songiil Budak Diler, "Genotoxicity of Aspartame," *Drug and Chemical Toxicology*, 2004, V 27, N 3: 257-268, http://cat.inist.fr/?aModele=afficheN&cpsidt=16108183.

64. "Chromosome," answers.com, http://www.answers.com/topic/chromosome.

65. C. Trocho, R. Pardo, I. Rafecas, J. Virgili, X. Remesar, J.A. Fernández-López and M. Alemany, "Formaldehyde Derived from Dietary Aspartame Binds to Tissue Components in Vivo," Universitat de Barcelona, Spain, 1998, http://www.presidiotex.com/barcelona/DISCUSSION/discussion.html.

66. Ronnie Cummins, "Hazards of Genetically Engineered Foods and Crops: Why We Need A Global Moratorium," *In Motion Magazine*, 29 August 1999, http://www.inmotionmagazine.com/geff4.html.

67. Ibid

68. Jeffrey M. Smith, *Seeds of Deception: Exposing Industry and Government Lies "*

69. Cummins, 1999.

70. Dr. Mercola, "Warning—GM Food Linked to Cancer," 8 March 2007, http://articles.mercola.com/sites/articles/archive/2007/03/08/warning----gm-food-linked-to-cancer.aspx.

71. Smith, 2003: 54, 64, 65.

72. Mica Rosenberg, "Mexico farmers quietly plant banned GM corn," 7 March 2008, http://www.reuters.com/article/inDepthNews/idUSN0732845620080307.

73. Leonard G. Horowitz, DMD, *Emerging Viruses: AIDS & Ebola, Nature, Accident or Intentional?*, Tetrahedron, Inc., 1996, p. 484, 485.

74. "Polio Vaccine," 4 June 2009, http://www.economicexpert.com/a/Polio:Vaccine.htm.

75. Horowitz, 1996, p. 493.

76. Ibid, p. 488, 492.

77. Jeffrey M. Smith, "American Academy of Environmental Medicine Calls for Immediate Moratorium on All Genetically Modified Foods," opednews.com, 19 May 2009, http://www.opednews.com/articles/American-Academy-of-Enviro-by-Jeffrey-M-Smith-090519-809.html.

78. Ibid.

79. Ibid.

80. Ibid.

81. Ibid.

82. Ibid.

83. Smith, 2003, p. 11.

84. Smith, 2009.

85. Ibid.

86. Ibid.

87. Ibid.

88. Ibid.

89. Ibid.

90. Ibid.

91. Kate Spinner, "As Africanized honeybees settle in Florida, residents need to be cautious, experts warn," 3 April 2006, http://www.aafricankillerbee.com/gpage6.html.

92. Ibid.

93. "Colony collapse disorder," Wikipedia, the Free Encyclopedia, http://en.wikipedia.org/wiki/Colony_Collapse_Disorder.

94. Sara Solovich, "Bee Prepared," *Philadelphia Enquirer*, 30 July 1989, http://www.sarasolo.com/pi.html.

95. Smith, 2003, p. 45, 76, 106, 126, 157, 230.

96. "Phytoestrogens," http://www.soyonlineservice.co.nz/04phytoestrogens.htm.

97. Clark Grosvenor, "Hormones and Growth Factors in Milk," *Endocrine Reviews*, V. 14, N. 6, 1992.

98. U.S.D.A., "Phytochemical and Ethnobotanical Database," http://www.ars-grin.gov/cgi-bin/duke/farmacy2.pl.

99. Can-Lan Sun, Jian-Min Yuan, Kazuko Arakawa, Siew-Hong Low, Hin-Peng Lee and Mimi C. Yu, "Dietary Soy and Increased Risk of Bladder Cancer," Cancer Epidemiology Biomarkers & Prevention V. 11, pps.1674-1677, December 2002, http://cebp.aacrjournals.org/cgi/content/abstract/11/12/1674.

100. Kate Melville, "Estrogen May Fuel Lung Cancer Growth," 3 April 2000, http://www.scienceagogo.com/news/20000302190630data_trunc_sys.shtml.

101. Susan Conova, "Estrogen's Role in Cancer," Columbia University Health Sciences, http://www.cumc.columbia.edu/news/in-vivo/Vol2_Iss10_may26_03/index.html.

102. Clair Weaver, "Cancer warning on soy foods," The Sunday Telegraph, January 14, 2007, http://www.news.com.au/story/0,23599,21057611-421,00.html.

103. Howard F. Lyman with Glen Merzer, *Mad Cowboy: Plain Truth from the Cattle Rancher who Won't Eat Meat*, Scribner, 1998: 11-12.

104. L. Peter, Health Hazards and Safety Considerations, http://www.fao.org/docrep/004/x6518e/X6518E04.htm.

105. Ibid.

106. Ibid.

107. Ibid.

108. Ibid.

109. Life expectancy of a cow?, http://answers.yahoo.com/question/index?qid=20070527130136AAA8VSq.

110. L. Peter, year unknown.

111. T. Colin Campbell, PhD, Thomas M. Campbell II, The China Study: Startling Implications for Diet, Weight Loss and Long-Term Health, Benbella Books, Dallas, Texas, 2006, p 7, 22.

112. Ibid.

113. Ibid: 348-349.

114. Ibid: 6.

115. Ibid: 367-368.

116. David Biello, "Bringing Cancer to the Dinner Table: Breast Cancer Cells Grow Under Influence of Fish Flesh; Tests of river fish indicate their flesh carries enough estrogen-mimicking chemicals to cause breast cancer cells to grow," Scientific American, 17 April 2007, http://www.scientificamerican.com/article.cfm?id=bringing-cancer-to-dinner-table-breast-cancer-cells-grow-under-influence-fish-flesh.

117. "Bisphenol A," From *Wikipedia,* the free encyclopedia, http://en.wikipedia.org/wiki/Bisphenol_A.

118. "A Tale of Two Estrogens: BPA and DES," Breast Cancer Fund, http://www.breastcancerfund.org/site/c.kwKXLdPaE/b.3959141/k.337F/A_Tale_of_Two_Estrogens_BPA_and_DES.htm.

119. "Bisphenol A," From *Wikipedia.*

120. Ibid.

121. Paloma Alonso-Magdalena, Sumiko Morimoto, Cristina Ripoll, Esther Fuentes, Angel Nadal, "The Estrogenic Effect of Bisphenol A Disrupts Pancreatic β-Cell Function In Vivo and Induces Insulin Resistance," Universidad Miguel Hernández de Elche, Alicante, Spain; Instituto Nacional de Ciencias Médicas y Nutrición Salvador Zubirán, México City, México, *Environmental Health Perspectives*, V 114, N 1, January 2006, http://www.ehponline.org/members/2005/8451/8451.html.

122. Janette Brand-Miller, Susanna Holt, Dorota Pawlak, Joanna McMillan, "Glycemic index and obesity," *American Journal of Clinical Nutrition*, V 76, N 1: 281S-285S, July 2002, http://www.ajcn.org/cgi/content/abstract/76/1/281S.

123. Alonso-Magdalena, et. al., 2006.

124. "Bisphenol A," From *Wikipedia.*

125. A Tale of Two Estrogens: BPA and DES.

126. Ibid.

127. Ibid.

128. Rowan Hooper, "Top 11 compounds in US drinking water," New Scientist, 12 January 2009, http://www.newscientist.com/article/dn16397-top-11-compounds-in-us-drinking-water.html.

129. Maxine Wright-Walters, MSc., Conrad Volz, Dr.PH, MPH, "Municipal Wastewater Concentrations of Pharmaceutical and Xenoestrogens: Wildlife and Human Health Implications," University of Pittsburgh, 23 August 2007, http://74.125.155.132/search?q=cache:Lz7HAfmhnmkJ:www.chec.pitt.edu/Exposure_concentration_of_Xenoestrogen_in_pharmaceutical_and_Municipal_Wastewater__Finalpaper_8-23-07_DR.VOLZ%255B2%255D.doc+2000+water+supply+chemicals+memick+estrogen&cd=2&hl=en&ct=clnk&gl=us.

130. Dr. Mercola, "Tap Water Toxins: Is Your Water Trying to Kill You?," http://articles.mercola.com/sites/articles/archive/2009/02/05/tap-water-toxins-is-your-water-trying-to-kill-you.aspx.

131. Ibid.

132. Ibid.

133. Ibid.

134. Ibid.

135. Ibid.

136. Russell Blaylock, MD, "Why Fluoride Is Toxic," http://www.newsmaxstore.com/newsletters/blaylock/reports/Blaylock4_Fluoride.htm.

137. Ibid.

138. Ibid.

139. Ibid.

140. Ibid.

141. Jane Kay, "Around the House: Indoor air pollution, Home is where the hazard is: Indoor toxins may be worse for you than outdoor smog," San Francisco Chronicle, 19 May 2004, http://www.sfgate.com/cgi-bin/article.cgi?file=/chronicle/archive/2004/05/19/HOGDC6LU141.DTL.

142. Ibid.

143. Ibid.

144. Ibid.

145. Ibid.

Numerics

A

mints containing 53
molecular
    composition 67
    mass 68
motor neuron disease 41
multiple sclerosis 41
multipotent carcinogenic agent 19
muscle weakness 41
myasthenia gravis 41
name assigned by IUPAC 68
neuralgia 41
neurological
    complications 41
    disorders 62
neurotoxin and teratogen 44
no adverse effects in industry-funded studies 61
no brain tumors in industry-funded studies 19
numbness 44
obesity 37
peripheral neuropathy 41
pharmacokinetic profile, capsules versus solution 7
phenylalanine levels, capsules versus solution 7
poisoning 9
promotes cancer growth, metastasis 96
protruding eyes 31
rare disorders of nervous system 42
rebranding by Ajinomoto as AminoSweet ix
scientific name 68
sensitivity 61
sold
    in beverages in 1983 69
    in dry goods in 1981 69
solution form
    absorbed more completely than capsules, solids 94
    more potent than capsule form 7
source for my experiment 3
tolerance in healthy subjects 61
unstable in aqueous media 9
weight gain 71
women outnumber men with adverse effects 93
yellowing fur 26, 34
Aspartame Consumer Safety Network 53
Aspartame Information Center 12, 67
Aspartame, Physiology and Biochemistry 6
aspartame.net 77
aspartameexperiment.com 82, 91, 92
aspartic acid ix, 7, 9, 68, 71
Associated Press 69
Atenolol 115
atherosclerosis 70, 71
atrazine 102, 115
    ambystoma tigrinum virus (ATV) 102
    Americans consume large quantities yearly 102
    birth defects, deformities, breast, prostate cancer 101
    deformed genitalia 102

fungal, viral diseases 102
herbicide banned in EU 101
inhibits mitochondrial ATP production of sperm 102
interferes with cellular uptake of dopamine 102
lowers white blood cell count 102
mimics estrogen 102
produces infertility 102
suppresses immune system 102
attention-deficit disorder 41
Austin, Donald, MD 117
Australia 109
autolyzed yeast 71
average
    daily aspartame intake 11
    lifespan of monkey 94
    weight of rats 11
avian flu 108
azamethiphos 100

B

bacillus thuringiensis (Bt) toxin 106
bacteria, genetically engineered 104
Barbara Kantrowitz 69
Barbara Mullarkey 53
Battelle Memorial Institute 117
Bayer 113
beef industry 109
benzene 14
Bernadine Magnuson 21
Betty Martini, D.Hum x, 67, 103, 124, 127, 131, 134
Bhargava, Pushpa M., PhD 106
Biello, David 112
Bienvia 67
Bill Deagle MD 103
birth defects 44
    caused by herbicide atrazine 101
    phenylalanine 44
bisphenol A (BPA) 113
    affects hearts of women 114
    affects memory, learning, mood 114
    carcinogenic, neurotoxic, linked to obesity 113
    decline in semen quality in men 114
    early onset of puberty in girls 114
    endocrine disrupter 113
    increase in breast, prostate cancer 114
    insulin-resistant (type 2) diabetes 114
    interference with brain cell connections 114
    metabolic disorders 114
    mimics hormones 113
    neurobehavioral problems, ADHD 114
    obesity in children, adults 114
    permanently damages DNA of mice 114
    reducing exposure to 114
    uro-genital abnormalities in male animal babies 114

drugs
    affect elderly more 95
    companies test own 3
    understanding how they affect us in old age 95
drugs.com 98
DSM Nutritional Products 22
Dupont 21, 22
duration 16
    of FDA accepted animal studies 14
    of my experiment 13, 14
    until spontaneous death of rats 4
dystonia 43
    dopa-responsive 41
    hereditary progressive 43

E

E. Coli, see Escherichia coli
E104 (quinoline yellow) 99
E133 (brilliant blue) 99
E621 (MSG) 99
E951 (aspartame) 67, 99
ears, ringing in 76
eau de cologne 76, 77
Echiverria, Santiago 78
Ecological Applications 102
Eli Lilly 22
Elsas, Louis, MD 44
embalming fluid 78
EMS (eosinophilia myalgia syndrome) 104
endocrine
    disorders 41
    system 49
Endocrine Society 114
Environmental Protection Agency (EPA) 77, 98, 101
Environmental Science & Technology 119
eosinophilia myalgia syndrome (EMS) 104
Epstein-Barr infection 46
Equal 67, 71, 95
Equal Measure 67
Equal Sugar Lite 67
Escherichia coli (E. Coli) bacteria
    from human and animal excrement 103
    genetically engineered, used to create
        L-aspartic acid in aspartame 103
        L-phenylalanine in aspartame 103
    most common species of fecal bacteria 103
    strain 85 synthesizes most L-aspartic acid 103
    synthesized chemicals may contain waste of 103
estrogen
    atrazine mimics 102
    breast, endometrial, uterine cancers 108
    carcinogenic 108, 112, 116
    dairy 108

dyslipidemia, disruption of lipids (fats) in blood 113
    hypertension 113
    in fecal matter in meat, poultry meals 110
    in tap water 115
    indeterminate genders in fish 112
    insulin resistance 113
    makes male fish indistinguishable from females 112
    mimicked by surfactants, flame retardants, halogenated hydrocarbons 115
    pharmaceutical 115, 116
    sex reversals, intersex individuals, alterations in mating, lack of gonadal maturation 116
    soy 108
    type 2 diabetes mellitus 113
Estrone 115
ethanol 76, 77, 78, 79
    antidote to methanol 78
    found in fruits, vegetables 78
    not in aspartame 78
Europe 107
European bees 107
European Food Information Council 22
European Ramazzini Foundation (ERF) 19
European Union 101
euthanized pets 109
Evangelista, Arthur M. 43, 124
evolutionary genetics 16
excitotoxins 70, 71, 72
    promote cancer growth, metastasis 96
Excitotoxins, the Taste that Kills ix
experiment, duration of my 13
experimental
    group, number of rats in 4
    protocol 3
    setup 1
exposure to multiple toxins, environmental stressors 99
extreme anger 48
Exxon 22
eyes
    bleeding 46, 47, 49, 53
    blind spot 53
    blindness 53
    blurred vision 56, 77
    disorders 62
    infections 46, 47, 48
    macular degeneration 53
    obliterative vasculitis 53
    protruding 51
    retina
        detachment of 51
        holes in 51
    sight problems 75
    tiny veins breaking 53
    warping 53

Russell Blaylock, MD ix, x, 7, 41, 42, 49, 70, 71, 96, 98, 118, 121, 122, 124, 125, 126, 129, 132, 136
rxlist.com 95

S

Sabin, Albert 105
sacrificing animals 13
Safe and Adequate Daily Intake (SAI) of fluoride 97
Sakow, Norm, DC 8
Salk Institute 106
Samuels, Jack 71, 95, 98
San Diego 115
San Diego State University 115
San Francisco Chronicle 119
Sanecta 67
sarcoma 102
    soft tissue 100
SARS 108
scalp feeling tight 58
Schenck, Susan 73
Schubert, David, PhD 106
science, consensus 91
Searle and Company, G.D., see G.D. Searle and Company
Seeds of Deception 104
seizures 5
serotonin 49
Shell Oil 22
shellac 76
Showa Denko 104
simian virus 40 (SV40)
    causes cancer 105
    causes hamsters to grow tumors 105
    remains active in Sabin vaccines 105
Sjogren's syndrome 41
skin 54
    lesions 54
    open ulcers 53
    problems 27, 32, 53, 62, 76
    rash 76
    red scaly patches, Psoriasis 76
    separating from body 56
sleep
    apnea 41
    paralysis 41
    problems 49
Slovak, Robert 116
small stove fuel 76
Smith
    Deborah, PhD 107
    Jeffrey 104, 106
snowdrop plant 104

sodium
    caseinate 71
    nitrate 102
Soffritti, Morando, MD, see Morando Soffritti, MD
soft tissue sarcoma 100
Soil Association 99
soil bacterium, bacillus anthrax 106
Southern Nevada Water Authority 115
soy
    adverse effects 73, 108
    bladder cancer 108
    dangers 109
    genetically engineered 106
    lung cancer 108
    post-menopausal bleeding 108
soybeans 108
Spain 103
spasmodic torticollis 42, 45
Spencer, P.S. 23
spontaneous deaths of animals 4
Sprague-Dawley rats 16, 19
stabilization of obesity epidemic 69
Stargel, W. Wayne, Pharm.D. 61
stealth viruses 105
    from African monkeys 105
    missing genes 105
    persistent infections 105
step-father, death of 95
Stockholm, Sweden 100, 102
stomach upset 76
studies
    104-Week Toxicity Study in the Mouse 4
    2,500 show vitamin D, cancer-prevention link 101
    46-Week Oral Toxicity—Hamster 4
    adequate methodology needed 3
    adverse effects found in independently funded 1
    all human studies short term 16
    animal, aspartame in dry food 94
    animal, in vitro, of green tea 96
    aspartame
        crystals clump or fall to bottom of food mix 94
        in milk ingested by monkeys 94
        primate study by Harry Waisman, MD 94
        solution more potent than capsules 7
    bisphenol A (BPA), estrogen 17β-estradiol (E2) 113
    black tea, high fluoride levels 97
    chlorinated water, bladder, rectal cancers 116
    developmental assessment of infant macaques 4
    double-blind human, aspartame in capsules 94
    drug companies test own drugs 3
    drug tests don't reflect real world 3
    estrogen produces eggs in male fish gonads 112
    fish extracts cause breast cancer 112

GE potatoes
    damage vital organs, immune systems 104
    found poisonous to mammals 104
human
    aspartame in capsules 7
    many lasted one week or less 95
    not continued through older years 95
    performed for less than 1% average lifetime 95
    some lasted 24 hours 95
identifying diffused carcinogenic risks 3
lack in elderly human population 95
low-protein diets inhibit initiation of cancer 111
mega experiments 3, 10, 14, 19
mirroring human condition 14
monkey seizures, death 94
MSG causes obesity 70
my results contradict aspartame industry 2
no adverse effects found in industry-funded 1
pesticides carcinogenic 100
pharmaceutical industry-sponsored 16
protocols insufficient for diffused carcinogens 3
sacrificing animals at 110 weeks 14
Soffritti
    observes rats until death 94, 95
tap water, pharmaceuticals, hormonally
    active chemicals 115
The China Study 111
toxicity of aspartame 17
water fluoridation increases cancer 117
sugar 58
Sugar Twin Plus 67
sugarless gum 45
suicide attempts 49
sulfallate 100
sulfamethoxazole 115
sunlight requirement for vitamin D 101
Sunoco 113
surfactants, flame retardants, halogenated hydrocarbons
    mimic estrogens 115
Suzuki, David, PhD 107
SV40, see simian virus 40
Sweden 100, 102
Sweet Misery 5
Sweetex 67
sweets, hunger for 71
swine flu 104, 108
synergistic effects, xenoestrogen mixtures 116
synthetic
    chemicals 13
    sweetener 67, 95

T

T. Colin Campbell, PhD 111
T4+ T cells 96

Taiwan 111
tap water 115, 116
TCEP 115
tea
    accumulates aluminum 98
    accumulates fluoride 97
    black
        from more mature leaves 97
        more fluoride than white or green tea 97
        most processed 98
    brick
        from oldest leaves 97
        highest fluoride content 97
        shaped into bricks 97
    camelia sinensis 96
    decaffeinated, high fluoride content 98
    green
        from fully developed leaves 97
        inhibits
            head, neck, pancreatic cancer 96
            leukemia, cervical, prostate cancer 96
        more processed than white tea 98
        organic, fluoride free 98
        reduces risk of
            breast, ovarian cancer 96
            gastro-intestinal, colon, lung cancer 96
            skin cancer 96
    helps protect against MSG 96
    iced, high fluoride content 98
    lemon precipitates aluminum from 98
    older crops, fewer beneficial phytochemicals 98
    white
        least fluoride 97
        least processed 98
        organic 97
temperature
    aspartame breaks down under high 6
    controlled in the body using serotonin 49
Terry Burnhan, PhD 16
testicular
    cancer 116
    dysgenesis 116
textured protein 71
The Bressler Report x, 6, 7
The Burdock Group 21
The Clinical Evaluation of a Food Additive
    Assessment of Aspartame 7, 95
The New York Times 111
The NutraSweet Company 6, 22, 61
The Philippines 106
The Raw Food Factor 73
theanine
    improved mood, learning ability, reduced anxiety,
        blood pressure, cholesterol, weight 96
    in tea, competitive antagonist to glutamate 96

thinning fur 32, 55, 56, 57, 62
thirst 56
Thomas Pynchon 81
Tibetans, brick tea, dental fluorosis 97
Tinnitus 76
tiny veins in eyes breaking 53
tiredness 56
tobacco smoke 119
torticollis 42, 45
Tourette's syndrome 41
Toxic Substances Control Act 119
Traditional Medicinals 98
tremors 41
triazine herbicides, ovarian cancer 102
trihalomethanes (THMs) 116
    stillbirths, spontaneous abortions, congenital
        malformations 117
Trimethoprim 115
Tri-Sweet 67
Trocho study 58, 78, 103
truthinlabeling.org 71, 95
tryptophan 49
Tschanz, Christian, MD 7, 61
tumor
    promoters 100
    rate 91, 93
        67% among females 93
tumors
    appeared in last third of lifetimes 94
    control group 62
    female controls with 38, 39, 40
    females on aspartame with 24, 25, 26, 27, 28, 29, 30,
        31, 32, 33, 34
    males on aspartame with 34, 35, 36, 37, 38
Turkey 103
Twinsweet 22, 67
type-2 diabetes 70, 71
tyrosine 48, 49

U

U.S. Air Force, pilot problems with aspartame 45
U.S. Congress 117
U.S. Department of Agriculture (USDA) 78, 108
U.S. Environmental Protection Agency (EPA) 98,
113, 119
U.S. Food and Drug Administration (FDA) x, 18, 98, 105,
121, 122, 124, 127
    77% of aspartame complainants are female 93
    92 documented aspartame symptoms 67
    acceptable daily intake (ADI) of aspartame 12
    consumer complaints about aspartame 53
    does not supervise drug tests 3
U.S. National Institutes of Health (NIH) 114

U.S. National Toxicology Program (NTP) 114
UC San Diego School of Medicine 101
ulcerated skin 53
Ulrike Peters 24
unauthorized website 81, 85, 91, 92
Universities Associated for Research and Education in
    Pathology (UAREP) 4
University of California, San Diego 101
University of Liverpool 99
University of Louisville Medical School 23
University of North Carolina at Chapel Hill 70
University of Pittsburgh 108, 112, 115
University of Southern California 105
University of Western Ontario 104
unsteadiness 41
Upjohn 22
upset stomach 76
urination, frequent 76
USDA Phytochemical and Ethnobotanical Database 96

V

vaccines
    American-made, contaminated by viruses 105
    Orimune live polio 105
varnish 76
vegan diet 73
Velsicol Chemical 22
verbal aggression 75
Victor Cecilioni, MD 117
vinyl chloride 14
violent criminal behaviors 49
viral diseases, atrazine 102
viral promoter, see Cauliflower Mosaic Virus
viruses
    contaminate American-made vaccines 105
    cytomegaloviruses
        herpes, infects man, monkey, other animals 105
        in monkeys imported for vaccine production 105
    destroy cells, unrecognized by immune system 105
    dormant monkey 105
    stealth 105
        cause persistent infections 105
        from African monkeys 105
        missing genes 105
visceral fat 72
vitamin D
    2,500 studies show cancer-prevention link 101
    D3 supplementation 101
    depressed blood levels make IGF-1 more active 112
    sunlight exposure required 101
Volz, Conrad 112
vomiting 77

W

X

Y

Z

13521451R00094